# Juran Institute

Juran Institute, a pioneer and world leader in managing for quality, was founded by Joseph M. Juran. The Institute provides resources, consulting, training, and comprehensive support to client organizations in the United States and internationally. The organization works with clients in large and small organizations and in diverse settings that include health care, financial services, publishing, manufacturing, high tech, aerospace, government, law, transportation, and others.

In health care, Juran Institute is actively involved in helping a wide range of organizations lay the foundation for long-term continuous quality improvement (CQI) of all operations, functions, and processes. Juran Institute has been a charter sponsor of the National Demonstration Project on Industrial Quality Control and Health Care Quality, and senior staff members continue to provide leadership, consultation, and instruction to individual organizations and systems, groups within organizations, and professional associations throughout health care's many arenas.

For more information contact:

Juran Institute
Eleven River Road
P.O. Box 811
Wilton, CT 06897–0811

Telephone: (203) 834–1700
FAX: (203) 834–9891

# The Juran Prescription

Kathleen Jennison Goonan, M.D.

· · · · · · · · · · · · · · · · · · · · · · · · · · · · · · · ·

Foreword by
A. Blanton Godfrey

# The Juran Prescription

Clinical Quality Management

Jossey-Bass Publishers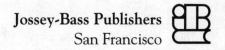
San Francisco

Substantial discounts on bulk quantities of Jossey-Bass books are available to corporations, professional associations, and other organizations. For details and discount information, contact the special sales department at Jossey-Bass Inc., Publishers. (415) 433–1740; Fax (800) 605–2665.

For sales outside the United States, please contact your local Paramount Publishing International Office.

 Manufactured in the United States of America on Lyons Falls Pathfinder Tradebook. This paper is acid-free and 100 percent totally chlorine-free.

### Library of Congress Cataloging-in-Publication Data

Goonan, Kathleen Jennison.
    The Juran prescription : clinical quality management / Kathleen
  Jennison Goonan.— 1st ed.
      p.   cm.—(Joint publication in the Jossey-Bass health and
  management series)
    Includes bibliographical references and index.
    ISBN 0-7879-0096-6 (alk. paper)
    1. Medical care—Quality control. 2. Total quality management.
  I. Title. II. Series: Jossey-Bass health series. III. Series:
  Jossey-Bass management series.
    [DNLM: 1. Juran, J. M. (Joseph M.), date. 2. Total Quality
  Management—organization & administration. 3. Quality Assurance,
  Health Care—organization & administration.  W 84.1 G659j 1995]
  RA399.A1G66   1995
  362.1'068'5—dc20
  DNLM/DLC
  for Library of Congress                                          94-46126
                                                                        CIP

FIRST EDITION
*HB Printing*    10 9 8 7 6 5 4 3 2 1

# Contents

• • • • • • • • • • • • • • • • • • • • • • • • • • • • •

# List of Tables, Figures, and Exhibits

· · · · · · · · · · · · · · · · · · · · · · · · · · · · · · · · · · ·

## Tables

## Figures

# Exhibits

# Foreword

· · · · · · · · · · · · · · · · · · · · · · · · · · · · · ·

Over the past eight years there has been a rapid evolution in the use of total quality management methods in health care. At first, health care organizations saw quality management in much the same way as manufacturing industries had viewed their efforts. Total quality management was just a way of taking unnecessary costs out of the system. With cost pressures from all sides—the payers, the public, and competitors—it was perhaps natural that this would be the case. It was also much easier to translate what was being done in industry to the administrative processes of the hospital or health maintenance organization (HMO) than it was to clinical processes. These business processes were in many ways similar; similar in their operation and similar in being riddled with waste and non-value-added steps.

Many health care organizations had paid little attention to the administrative side: inventories were huge, billing processes cumbersome and costly, expensive equipment and facilities were grossly underutilized, and information systems were embryonic and unconnected. The opportunities for quick improvements were legion, and staffs were more than ready to make fast changes. Many organizations made rapid improvements and moved significant sums to the bottom line.

The other side of quality, the customer side, had been for years the focus of physicians, nurses, and health care administrators. Years of outcomes research led to new medicines, new procedures, and new technologies. Recent studies on patient-focused care had created new understanding and even new organizational structures. Clinical pathways were developed for many diagnostic related groups and were being used to increase both efficiency and effectiveness. An entire quality assurance science was developed to monitor, report, and act on all violations of good medical practice.

It was far less clear what modern quality management philosophies, concepts, techniques, and tools had to offer the clinical side of care. A few pioneers saw the possibilities. They saw that while health care had made great strides in understanding patient needs and creating new processes for meeting these needs, for the most part these understandings were still based on the views of physicians, nurses, and administrators and not on those of patients, patients' families, or payers.

They also saw that the entire quality assurance methodology had become obsessed with finding and fixing blame rather than changing the care processes that allowed errors to happen. Industrial companies fighting globally for survival had developed tremendous passions for finding the true root causes of problems and removing the causes permanently. This passion was missing in health care organizations. The same philosophies, concepts, and tools used by these companies to drive quality upstream in the processes and focus on prevention rather than inspect-and-fix could also revolutionize health care.

Kathleen Jennison Goonan, M.D. was one of the revolutionary pioneers. Early on in her career she saw how many of the traditional measurements used in even leading HMOs were not based on any thorough understanding of customer needs. She saw that many health care organizations did not even have clear definitions of who the customers were. She worked at first to create these understandings and to develop the measurements needed to track how an organization was really doing in the eyes of its customers.

But Dr. Goonan saw other possibilities too. She saw how these same modern quality management ideas and tools could be used to actually improve the outcomes of medical interventions. By understanding the entire care process, she could see where to make informed changes that not only would change the cost of care but also would significantly improve the quality of care.

In the past few years many others have also seen these possibilities. Where only a few years ago one had to search hard to find clinical quality improvement examples, now almost every journal and report is full of such stories. Dr. Goonan has captured many of these examples in this book and carefully explained not just *what* was done but *how* it was done. These examples, coupled carefully with the theory and tools, give a glimpse of what can be achieved and how some organizations are already making substantial breakthroughs in care.

The practical nature of this book is illustrated by the chapter, "Implementing Quality Management in Clinical Settings," by Robert B. Halder, M.D. In this chapter Dr. Halder uses his extensive experience as a physician, a CEO of a major hospital, and a consultant to a number of leading organizations to define a step-by-step roadmap for implementing total quality management (or continuous quality improvement). He not only defines each step in detail, he also gives specific actions the senior clinical leadership of the organization must take. His liberal use of examples makes it easy to understand just what should be done and how it should be done. Those just starting in applying modern quality management to clinical care will find this chapter an invaluable guide. Those already well under way can use this chapter as a checklist to review what steps they may have overlooked and to gain some insight into how to accelerate the pace or to remove the barriers to success.

There are many things that distinguish this book. The first is Dr. Goonan's emphasis on the process of providing care. She reviews the nature of variation in medical practice and stresses the importance of process capability. She addresses head-on the hard issues such as measurement. Her care in defining the steps for quality improvement in clinical quality provides a much needed primer for success.

Most readers will find many revelations in the chapter on quality planning. Designing optimal care either through clinical practice guidelines or patient-focused care delivery requires concepts and tools beyond basic problem-solving methods. Dr. Goonan provides an in-depth guide to systematic quality planning with a step-by-step approach that includes everything from establishing goals to deploying and evaluating the delivery process. Her use of case studies and examples provides the clarity needed for one to apply quality planning in a clinical setting.

All organizations—industrial, service, and health care—are continually inventing and reinventing new means for improving quality and lowering costs. What we know today is far greater than what we knew even a few years ago. And yet, many organizations are still struggling to apply these new ideas quickly to the clinical areas. *The Juran Prescription* provides us with a guide. The book's explanations, examples, and case studies should accelerate the pace of implementation for any organization.

*March 1995*                                    A. Blanton Godfrey
*Wilton, Connecticut*                              Chairman & CEO
                                                  Juran Institute, Inc.

# Preface

· · · · · · · · · · · · · · · · · · · · · · · · · · · · · · · · · ·

The social and economic environment in which practitioners care for patients changes daily. Numerous pressures drive clinicians to learn new management skills: process and outcome measurement, pathway and guideline development, epidemiological thinking, variation analysis, capitation, conflict negotiation, and the list goes on. Purchasers and the body politic expect health care organizations to identify, measure, improve continuously, and report publicly outcomes of care that meet yet-to-be-specified standards of quality and cost effectiveness. Many practitioners feel pressed to implement sweeping changes within their practices, hospitals, and managed-care organizations in order to survive professionally. Few practitioners have had the opportunity to learn the management skills necessary to be confident and successful during this transition.

Increasing numbers of health care organizations adapt by applying a variety of management strategies and techniques to help them succeed in this new, highly competitive environment. One world-renowned school of management, known as total quality management (TQM), stems from the work of Joseph M. Juran. Juran is the author of *Juran on Quality by Design, Juran on Planning for Quality,* and *Juran's Quality Control Handbook* and has received more than thirty awards for his innovations in quality control. TQM is based on the experiences of scores of organizations and hundreds of managers. Juran provides universal and practical wisdom on how to design and implement an organizational system for quality. Health care organizations began applying Juran's teachings in the late 1980s, and many organizations are thriving today as a result. All have learned important lessons worth sharing with others. Ironically, Juran's teachings overlap with a number of innovations in health care delivery, including outcomes measurement, guidelines for practice, reengineering, and patient-focused care. At its core, TQM offers clinical leaders a framework within which to organize all of these important initiatives.

## Audience and Purpose of This Book

This book is intended primarily for clinicians and clinical administrators who want to acquire knowledge and skills that will help them play a leadership role in this new environment. These new "subspecialists" must guide their colleagues and organizations toward achieving outstanding clinical outcomes and patient satisfaction in the context of continual learning, performance improvement, and documented value. Most practitioners do not have the time or the inclination to attend conferences or distill the literature for their own medical specialty, much less for quality management. This book is written for my colleagues, respectfully aware of the time constraints and pressures they face.

The purpose of the book is to offer a comprehensive overview of concepts, tools, and techniques useful to clinicians and managers. It surveys the breadth of knowledge and skills necessary for clinician leaders to master. It is not intended to provide proficiency in all these areas, rather to establish a foundation for continuing self-education and learning. The Juran Institute and many other educational resources offer a wide variety of training opportunities in quality management for health care professionals. Wherever possible, resources for further study are referenced. Descriptions of the clinical applications of TQM come from direct observations of organizations over the last eight years, including Intermountain Health Care, Uni-Health America, Kaiser Permanente, the Mayo Clinic, Sun Health, Harvard Community Health Plan, Blue Cross and Blue Shield of Massachusetts, and many more hospitals, group practices, and academic medical centers.

In sum, this book scans the myriad solutions being promoted and ties them into a logical and concise framework. It identifies the practical steps individuals and organizations can take to build their quality program. The prescription is built on Juran's teachings and the experience of clinician leaders in applying these teachings to managing patients, hospitals, HMOs, and managed-care organizations for eight years.

There are innumerable examples of management fads and gurus that have come and gone. Clinicians are reluctant to fall prey to the claims of magic bullets. I share this concern. But the fear of fads notwithstanding, there are skills, strategies, and techniques we can use to make practicing medicine more successful and worthwhile.

## Overview of the Contents

Chapter One distills the motivating political and economic challenges that create the need for new skills among clinician leaders. It lays out the basic elements of a comprehensive and mature quality system for any health care organization to succeed in today's environment. Chapter Two reviews the fundamental concepts and principles of quality management and their applicability to clinical practice into the future. "Why bother to master a field that sounds like jargon?" clinicians often ask. The answer is simple: because it can help optimize the care to patients *and* help organizations succeed in today's marketplace. Although examples appear throughout the book, Chapter Three describes in detail several stories of using the TQM approaches and tools in clinical settings from start to finish.

Juran identified three basic managerial processes or activities that must be in place within organizations that manage their quality, outcomes, satisfaction, loyalty, and cost; the next three chapters describe them. Chapter Four explores the tools and techniques needed to analyze inpatient and ambulatory practice patterns. It surveys the approaches to reducing unwanted variation that work well with clinicians and respect their individual professionalism. Chapter Five, on planning and designing care processes, surveys the tools and techniques proving useful for designing clinical care as well as entire delivery programs. It touches on patient-focused care and reengineering. Chapter Six explores the strategies useful for improvement project teams and the lessons learned from the organizations that have used them.

Chapter Seven looks at how clinical organizations can develop strategies, goals, and targets that coordinate this array of (expensive) activities and optimize results. Chapter Eight was written by Robert B. Halder, M.D., senior vice president at the Juran Institute. It describes an implementation roadmap based on the experience of many consultants and organizations using the Juran approach. The concluding chapter analyzes whether TQM offers a quick fix or a new lifestyle, one that requires self-discipline but offers long-term success.

## Acknowledgments

I want to thank many people who contributed knowledge to this book. First and foremost, my greatest respect for and gratitude to Joseph Juran. Had he been a physician rather than an engineer, he might have considered subspecializing in surgery, psychiatry, or primary care. Surgery would appeal to him because of his pragmatism and attention to design of solutions, psychiatry because of his awareness of personal development and the dynamics of relationships, and primary care because of his attentiveness to the continuum of experiences and the complexity of systems.

I also want to thank Bob Halder for writing Chapter Eight. Robert B. Halder, M.D., Rear Admiral, Medical Corps, U.S. Navy (retired), is senior vice president of Juran Institute, Inc. At the institute, Halder works closely with the senior management of our major health care organizations to develop and implement TQM systems. He also provides leadership in health care quality on a national and international level.

Halder had a distinguished career in the U.S. Navy as a senior executive and practicing ophthalmologist. He has experience as a clinician, medical staff leader, and chief operating officer. During his several years as a chief executive officer, including three years leading the Navy's largest hospital, he became recognized for implementing a successful managed and coordinated care program.

William Van Faasen and Joe Avellone, M.D., chief executive officer and chief operating officer, respectively, of Blue Cross and Blue Shield of Massachusetts, create an atmosphere where change and innovation can flourish. They supported the writing of this book.

Other major contributors include Maureen Bisognani, Chip Caldwell, and John Early, senior vice presidents at the Juran Institute. I also want to express my gratitude and admiration to my colleagues Turner Bledsoe, John Collins, Jan Cook, Richard Cornell, Michele Di Palo, Ann Marie Duquette, Harmon Jordan, Matt Kelliher, John Mason, and Pam Siren. Their tireless hours and endless creativity have allowed me to learn and grow as a quality professional. A special thanks to Brent James for all the years of thinking through these challenging issues together.

*March 1995*                          Kathleen Jennison Goonan, M.D.
*Boston, Massachusetts*

# The Author

. . . . . . . . . . . . . . . . . . . . . . . . . . . . . . . . . . . .

Kathleen Jennison Goonan, M.D., is director of medical policy, evaluation, and improvement for Blue Cross and Blue Shield of Massachusetts, where she is responsible for developing and coordinating clinical quality management activities for all indemnity and managed-care plans. Dr. Goonan was director of the Quality Indicators Program for Harvard Community Health Plan until 1992. In addition to being an instructor with the National Demonstration Project and now the Institute for Healthcare Improvement, she has been an associate of the Juran Institute since 1992 and lectures nationally on clinical quality management.

Dr. Goonan completed her internship and residency (1982–1985) as well as a research fellowship in general medicine at the Massachusetts General Hospital. She remained on staff there until 1989 and served on the Internal Medicine Department Quality Assurance Committee from 1987 to 1989. Her academic publications are in the area of quality measurement and incentives affecting physician practice patterns.

She is an honors graduate of the University of California, Santa Cruz; a graduate of the University of California, Davis, Medical School; and a member of the Alpha Omega Alpha Medical Honor Society. In 1982 she served as president of the American Medical Student Association in Washington, D.C.

# The Juran Prescription

# 1

New Skills for
Clinical Leaders

This chapter reviews the drivers for change that are motivating
clinicians to learn a new management approach and presents
the components of a comprehensive system to achieve cost-effective
quality care for patients and purchasers.

## Drivers of Reform

The rapid and dramatic growth of health care costs is viewed as
a major threat to the well-being of the U.S. economy as a whole.
In just the past thirty years, health care expenditures have risen
from less than 6 percent to nearly 14 percent of the total gross
domestic product. This fundamental shift has created a number
of forces driving health care leaders and managers to seek new
management skills.

The changes occurring in health care are known to anyone reading this book. The forces distill into a simple list: radical changes
in *payment* mechanisms and incentives, the resulting drive toward
vertical and horizontal *integration*, ever-increasing demand for
*accountability* on performance, and the net result, dramatic expectations of clinical leaders and *management* (see Figure 1.1). Successful clinicians and administrators will respond with new
leadership approaches and management skills.

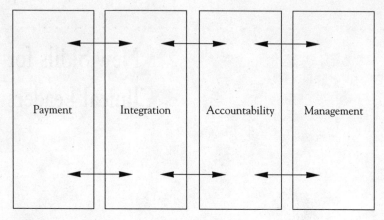

Figure 1.1.  Drivers for Change.

Consider first the fundamental shift in financing from cost-plus reimbursement to risk sharing, which has resulted in radically different incentives for hospitals, physicians, and other providers. Since the inception of medical insurance and entitlement programs during the 1960s, clinicians have been largely insulated from the ethical dilemma of assessing the cost-benefit of their actions. Prospective payment, capitation, and other risk-sharing arrangements intended to rein in health care cost inflation radically change clinician and institutional incentives. Clinicians can no longer ignore questions of cost effectiveness of interventions.

Under these new payment arrangements, practitioners and institutions have incentives to scrutinize each test or intervention that goes into the care of individual patients. For example, the Health Care Financing Administration (HCFA) experiment with Medicare bundled payment (all professional, institutional, and ancillary fees combined into one global fee) for the total care of coronary bypass surgery patients is generally considered a success, in terms of cost savings and quality of care (Cafasso, 1992; Winslow, 1992). It has inspired HCFA and other purchasers to create similar payment mechanisms for other procedures such as cataract extraction. For many hospitals, particularly those in highly competitive markets such as California (Campbell, 1993a), Minnesota (Stump, 1993), and Massachusetts, the trend is toward prospective payment for the total episode of illness by bundling the physician, ancillary, and institutional fees into one highly competitive price.

Experimentation with payment strategies is expected to grow dramatically in the next decade (Bader, 1993a). Finding the proper balance between incentives to provide care, as under fee for service, and incentives to withhold care, as under capitation, is the major challenge facing managed-care clinician leaders in the 1990s. Potentially, the best interests of patients and their needs for coordinated care will be served. But the risk of incentivizing undertreatment is undeniable. These changes in reimbursement drive horizontal integration and new dynamics between doctor and hospital, doctor and managed-care organization or payer, and even clinician and clinician. If managed properly, they foster collaboration around the continuum of care for episodes of illness and cohorts of patients. If managed poorly, they lead to conflict, waste, and fragmentation of care.

Reimbursement reform also drives vertical integration of delivery systems. Vertical integration refers to systems with explicit contractual or ownership arrangements that provide for services across the spectrum of settings and institutions—ambulatory, acute care, rehabilitative, and home care. Natural economies of scale and industry consolidation drive this integration. Achieving coordinated care for populations within these complex delivery systems requires leadership and management expertise at a level not present in most health care organizations today. Organizations that respond creatively to this driver will gain a competitive advantage.

The third driver to increase medical management skills is the demand for accountability. Purchasers and payers expect documentation of the value of health care services provided to their employees and insured populations (Relman, 1988, p. 1220). In an effort to understand and justify increasing expenditures and become prudent buyers, purchasers are coordinating efforts to judge the worth of the health care they pay for. Some sectors of health care, such as rehabilitation and behavioral health, have lived with this expectation for years because of variable health insurance benefits and the pressure to justify coverage of their services. Today, all health care specialties are expected to justify the cost-benefit of their interventions. This requires health care leaders to have a strategy and methods to measure and account for the value of the services their organizations provide, without adding to the overall administrative cost of health care. Moreover, purchasers take this expectation one step further and require documentation of continual improvement of cost effectiveness and outcomes over time.

These three drivers—payment incentives, organizational integration, and accountability—translate into global demand for medical managers to lead with new vision, strategy, and techniques. Clinician leaders need a systematic approach to transform a fee-for-service cottage industry into well-integrated, cost-efficient delivery systems achieving optimal outcomes with documented improvement in performance over time. Admittedly, this is no small task. The next section describes the fundamental elements that must be in place to successfully overcome these challenges.

## A Quality System

Over the past forty years, Joseph Juran (1989) delineated the fundamental components of a comprehensive approach to the management of quality (Figure 1.2). He identified the required elements of a system to measure, improve, and design processes that consistently deliver optimal outcomes. He named his system *total quality management*, or *TQM*. The expression sounds strangely industrial to most clinicians; however, Juran's universal principles derive from applying the basic scientific method to scores of diverse industrial and professional endeavors. These same principles have been applied to hospitals (Gaucher and Coffey, 1993), health maintenance organizations (Jennison Goonan and Jordan, 1992), and health systems

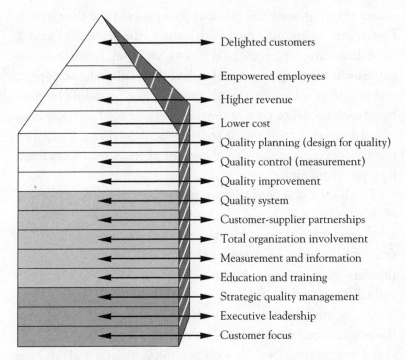

Figure 1.2. Total Quality Management.

(James, 1989). They have been adopted by numerous leading health care organizations since the late 1980s. Most of the early successes were in nonclinical "hotel service" or ancillary functions such as lab testing and radiology. Increasingly, health care organizations expand their efforts to include practitioners, patient care processes, and clinical outcomes (Campbell, 1993b; Kritchevsky and Simmons, 1991).

At the core of an organizational quality system is a well-defined and widely communicated approach to customers, leadership, and strategic quality planning (Juran, 1988). (In health care, "customers" are patients, employers, managed-care organizations, payers, and others.) Leaders within an organization must share a common understanding of their customers and their needs and expectations. They must formulate a vision for meeting or exceeding those needs that extends five to ten years into the future. For a hospital, this means knowing many things about your patients and their payers. First, it implies knowing the health status of the population served, their diagnostic mix, their health risks, and their health care use patterns. It also implies understanding their cultural, geographic, and insurance status. Finally, all this information should be combined with an astute view of the future of managed care and integrated delivery systems within an institution's market. All together, this type of strategic thinking about customers lays the foundation for a successful future.

There must also be significant investment in the development of new leaders and their skills. Traditionally, physician leadership roles were undervalued and undersupported. The principal role was to advocate for the self-interest of loosely affiliated individual practitioners. In today's environment, clinician leaders play a dramatically different role in relation to their clinician peers and other leaders within health care organizations. This requires investing in their professional development in a variety of ways. At a minimum, they need training in skills such as clinical process and outcome measurement, practice pattern analysis, clinical practice improvement techniques, guideline implementation, applied research methods, finance negotiation, and conflict resolution.

A third component of the foundation for a quality system is a comprehensive strategic planning process that identifies the goals, targets, and tactics to achieve the organization's vision. This is a critical responsibility for the leadership of any organization. For health care organizations, in the current state of tremendous flux, this becomes even more important. In a cost-plus health care market, clinicians were typically treated as customers of hospitals. After all, it was their decisions to admit patients and order various services that maintained hospitals financially. Within prospective payment, physicians must assume a leadership role as principal suppliers of health care. Today, physicians are expected to identify key diagnostic groups and processes of care that should be the focus of continuous measurement and improvement. These priorities must be set based on full knowledge and understanding of customer expectations and their accountability requirements. Once the priority areas of health care delivery have been identified, leaders must guide their peers in their efforts to measure process and outcomes of care, identify and replicate best practices, and document improvement in outcomes achieved for these patient populations.

The infrastructure for achieving delighted customers and increasing market share includes some functions already developed within many health care organizations (case management, quality assurance, patient-focused care, medical staff structure). Other functions must be added or changed to incorporate new approaches. Training takes a new form in a TQM organization. All staff and employees must be provided with new knowledge and skills. Most organizations develop both in-depth training programs for all staff and employees in quality measurement and management techniques, as well as "just-in-time" trainers, experienced continuous improvement team facilitators who can teach during project team meetings.

Information systems, typically designed to catalog charges and generate or process claims, must now become vehicles for tracking practice patterns and resource use to analyze and improve processes of care (Dick and Steen, 1991). They must provide real-time accounting of what actually occurs in patient care and what that care costs. These ever-increasing demands for actionable data and analytic capabilities necessitate new levels of sophistication from existing information systems. Data must be transformed into information that clinical leaders can use to help their colleagues identify and replicate optimal practice patterns. This is a very new and underdeveloped applied science that requires systems and information specialists who treat practitioners as their customers. Most leading health care organizations are investing heavily in the development of their information systems.

The fundamental work of managing quality and cost within an organization can be distilled into three basic quality management processes:

1. *Quality control* refers to ongoing measurement of key care processes and reduction of unintended and inappropriate variability in practice patterns. A major aspect of quality control is measurement and feedback of practice patterns. Critical pathways and decision algorithms are examples of tools designed to reduce variation that many organizations find helpful for some procedures and diagnoses.

2. *Quality planning* refers to a variety of tools and techniques to design care processes that are fundamentally different from the status quo. This might entail designing a patient-focused care approach or incorporating new knowledge about effective patient-care methods into a practice protocol, pathway, or guideline. Quality planning would be used to design a new care process or program targeting a particular patient population, such as women's health or cardiovascular disease. The quality planning approach is also used to overhaul or reengineer an existing process beset by problems.

3. *Quality improvement* is a set of measurement and change techniques that allow clinicians to evaluate and improve day-to-day practice and outcomes for cohorts of comparable patients. Improvement typically occurs project by project. Cross-functional work groups analyze how they currently care for patients and systematically identify how to improve outcomes by changing practice patterns.

These management processes, which Juran referred to as the "Juran Trilogy" (see Table 1.1), entail distinct yet related activities that can achieve optimal outcomes, cost effectiveness, satisfied customers, and increasing market share. Each relies on different tools and techniques and is appropriate for different problems.

Most health care organizations need to begin their TQM program by focusing on quality control activities. Ordinarily, the lack of actionable information on quality drives early-stage activity to focus on measurement. Customer reporting requirements can be another factor. Similarly, some organizations start by using quality control

Table 1.1. Managing for Quality.

| Quality Control | Quality Planning | Quality Improvement |
|---|---|---|
| Identify measurement needs | Identify current and future customers | Identify the needed improvement projects |
| Charter measurement team | Charter design team | Charter improvement project team |
| Evaluate actual performance | Determine customers' needs | Diagnose the causes |
| Compare actual performance to goals or benchmarks | Develop services responsive to customers' needs | Remedy the causes |
| Reduce unintended variation | Develop processes able to deliver service | Establish controls to hold the gains |
| | Transfer new process to clinicians | Identify opportunities to replicate the remedy |

tools such as pathways to demonstrate that unwanted variation in length of stay and charges can be reduced (see Chapter Four).

Typically, the second stage of TQM implementation in clinical care draws on the quality planning approach. Early measurement results often reveal great and inexplicable variation in many care processes and outcomes. This leads organizations to focus on practice guideline development (Chapter Five). The third quality management process is quality improvement (Chapter Six). In industrial settings, Juran recommends beginning TQM implementation with quality improvement projects. For clinical care, however, the lack of measurement and the magnitude of practice variation are so great as to make this difficult. Ultimately, every organization needs to roll out a quality management system tailored to its own unique circumstances. There is no one proper sequence for every organization.

In total, what Juran did in his writings was encapsulate the best teachings of many great scientists (Crosby, 1979; Donabedian, 1989; Walton, 1986) into a practical guide for action. The purpose of all of this infrastructure and activity is to achieve results:

- "Delighted" customers: patients, their families, and their employers or purchasers who recommend their health care providers to their friends and family.

- Better outcomes, including clinical, functional, satisfaction, and total cost of care measures.

- Lower cost for the same or better outcomes.

The magnitude of changes inherent in this prescription can be overwhelming. The remainder of this book looks at each of the basic elements of a quality system in greater depth.

# 2

· · · · · · · · · · · · · · · · · · · · · · · · · · · · · · · · · · · ·

# The Basic Physiology
# of Quality

This chapter summarizes quality management concepts as they apply to clinical practice and patient outcomes. Clinical applications of these methodologies are new and evolving, even in health care organizations that have already applied them in administrative processes. Clinicians are naturally skeptical about how this approach can assist in the care of patients and the success of clinical practice. Clinical training focuses on the care to individual patients. TQM applies to the doctor-patient relationship but also to the care delivered to populations of patients.

Learning the basic concepts of TQM is like learning basic physiology; both lay the knowledge base for other, more sophisticated skills. Some TQM concepts apply to clinical practice more readily than others. In many cases, concepts appear foreign when in fact the differences are largely related to terminology. Other concepts are new for clinicians and require more adaptation to apply in the clinical setting. More often than not, however, there is congruity between the traditional practice of medicine and TQM approaches to optimizing practice patterns and outcomes. Understanding and applying these universal management concepts open a wide array of opportunities for clinical organizations to succeed in today's environment.

## What Is Quality?

The first and most basic concept to master is a working definition of quality. Clinicians take an oath as professionals to provide quality care. Striving to do the best for individual patients is fundamental to a clinician's role and professional identity. However, to manage quality and value of health care services for whole populations over time, organizations need an operational definition of quality. That definition must be objective, measurable, and logical to practitioners, patients, and purchasers.

One definition that has proved useful in many quality management programs incorporates two simple concepts: features and freedom from deficiencies. These concepts are related but not opposites. Each is relevant to the challenge facing clinicians. Both must be addressed by organizations that survive the 1990s and beyond.

### Freedom from Deficiencies

Deficiencies abound in most organizations and professions; health care is no exception. When processes and people fail to achieve optimal results, they create potentially preventable patient suffering, wasted resources, unnecessary work for colleagues, and, in some cases, risk of litigation.

A clinical process deficiency can be defined as any avoidable error or unnecessary step in the prevention, diagnosis, and treatment of a health problem. Some examples include:

*Deficiencies*
•••••••••••••••••••••••••••••••••••••••••••

The time and resources that go into unnecessary care

The absence of necessary care

Wasted resources such as blood products or drugs

Preventable complications

Days in an acute-care hospital waiting for a nursing home bed

Practice patterns that deviate from recognized guidelines

Nosocomial infections

ER triage delays

Unplanned return to surgery

Post-op arrhythmia

Lost lab results

Premature discharge

Unnecessary tests or treatments

Deficiencies are costly to individual practitioners and organizations because they must be identified and corrected. They waste time and scarce resources. They may take the form of underservice within a prospective payment or capitated payment system or overservice in a fee-for-service payment system. People create "work-arounds"—means to accommodate defective processes that only add to the cost of care for patients.

Both unnecessary care and excessive care can be reduced when care processes perform optimally. Better patient outcomes result from care delivered without errors. While much is unproved about effectiveness and outcomes, organizations and individual practitioners are expected to demonstrate the use of tools (guidelines, profiling, feedback) to optimize practice patterns wherever possible.

Note that this definition of deficiencies encompasses both cost and quality. In the past, the medical profession has shied away from the complex ethical issues of considering cost-benefit of interventions for individual patients. Understandably, physicians prefer to avoid these thorny issues in the context of individual patient-care decisions. In Juran's definition of quality as it applies to clinical care, efficiency (resource use) and quality (performance) are viewed as aspects of the whole. Quality refers to error-free processes, including both wasted resources and suboptimal patient care.

Deficiencies, when present and known to patients, lead to dissatisfaction, distrust, and diminished loyalty. On the other hand, the absence of deficiencies does not necessarily lead to increased patient loyalty. Freedom from deficiencies is assumed by patients and only gets an organization to a grade C. When deficient care receives publicity, the loss of market share and reputation can be tremendous. Judging which deficiencies are critical to measure and eliminate is an important skill for medical managers to develop.

## Features

Features are defined as the aspects to patient care that attract patients, that distinguish one practitioner from another, or one hospital from the others. In the clinician's office, spending extra time with the patient above and beyond what is needed to provide professionally sound medical treatment is a concern in today's cost-conscious environment. It may not be necessary for optimal care but it may be a feature that many patients seek and value. Among the many examples of services are these:

*Service Features*

Unsolicited phone calls to the patient or family

Evening and weekend hours

Patient education videos

Affiliations with teaching hospitals

Services tailored to the particular needs of a diagnostic group

Case management

Pleasant waiting area

Focused-care programs

Patient reminder cards

Food access in room

Unlike deficiencies, building features into the process of care can lead to increased satisfaction and customer loyalty (see Table 2.1). It is important to pay attention to features because people continue to use the clinicians and facilities that meet their perceived needs and expectations. The better an organization understands patient expectations and provides services designed to meet those expectations, the greater the attraction to that organization. This can lead to community loyalty and higher revenues. However, providing more features can increase the costs of delivering care. Knowing which features to provide will help your organization thrive, but it takes careful planning.

Table 2.1.  What Is Quality?

|  | Features | Free from deficiency |
| --- | --- | --- |
| *Needs* | Right things | Done right |
| *Customer* | Satisfaction | Dissatisfaction |
| *Effect* | Income | Costs |
| *Higher quality costs* | More | Less |

### The Institute of Medicine's Definition

The Institute of Medicine appointed a seventeen-member committee in 1990 to define quality of care and quality assurance. After months of deliberations and input from hundreds of individuals, the following definition was arrived at: quality is "the degree to which health care services for individuals and populations increases the probability of desired health outcomes and is consistent with current professional knowledge of best practice" (Institute of Medicine, 1990). This definition incorporates the concept of freedom from deficiency but not necessarily the concept of features. Features are not required to meet the expectations of the profession but are an absolute necessity for success in a competitive marketplace. The following hypothetical case example highlights the distinctions between deficiencies and features.

### Case Example: A Diabetic Is Scheduled for Ophthalmologic Surgery

An eighteen-year-old insulin-dependent diabetic came in for a preoperative evaluation to the ambulatory medical evaluation unit. He was scheduled for a same-day vitrectomy the following morning at Excellent Eye Hospital (EEH). The medical unit is well regarded because it is staffed by respected internists from a neighboring teaching hospital. Patients are seen in the evening, with an average turnaround time of between forty-five and ninety minutes.

There are certain customs at EEH, such as taking the most labile diabetics first on the OR schedule and nurse practitioners who round on the postoperative patients. There are no explicit guidelines. Each patient has an individualized management plan and unique orders written by a medical unit consultant for the diabetes and other medical conditions.

The internist who evaluated the patient preoperatively noted that his diabetes is labile and, therefore, he should be one of the first cases of the day to ensure he is stabilized postoperatively. When the internist finished the evaluation and completed the preoperative and postoperative orders, she wrote for a fasting blood sugar (BS) measurement, as well as recovery room and 3:00 P.M. measurements. Her routine practice was to write for an evening measurement, but she forgot. As usual, she wrote for the patient to receive half his daily insulin dose in the morning, an IV of running glucose, and a sliding scale for insulin based on the postoperative BS measurement. She provided the patient with an explanation of what to expect over the next two days and gave him an information pamphlet that described the daily routines of EEH.

### A Break from Routine

For unknown reasons, this patient did not go to the operating room until midday. When he came to the recovery room it was already 3:30 P.M. so the nurses drew only one blood sugar; it was 225, a reasonable blood sugar for this patient. Because of the timing of his arrival to the recovery room, the nurse practitioners did not see him, assuming the medical unit physician would come by later. The physician, knowing the patient was to be an early case, assumed the nurse practitioners had checked on him postoperatively.

By midnight, the patient was urinating large volumes and complaining of increasing nausea and eye pain. The floor nurse assumed his nausea was from eye pain and gave him morphine. He received two more doses of narcotics before morning. At 6 A.M. he was found semicomatose, and the physician was called. A stat blood sugar measurement was 764. The patient was transferred to an acute-care hospital and stabilized over the next twelve hours. Fortunately, he recovered quickly without further complications.

The physician called the patient's mother to explain what had happened. The mother responded nonchalantly, blaming her son and his diabetes for the turn of events. The physician also called the boy's primary care physician, to alert him to the situation and to make him aware that the family might not be as supportive of the patient as might be hoped.

### Analysis

This example highlights both aspects of quality. There are issues of potential deficiency in the care to this patient as well as features in the care process that may or may not add to the value of being treated at Excellent Eye Hospital. On the deficiency side of the ledger, the physician made an error by not ordering an evening blood sugar. This led to inadequate data for clinical decision making. There were errors in judgment and interpretation of the patient's signs and symptoms. There was the failure to check a blood sugar in a diabetic with high urine volumes and vomiting.

With respect to features, the ambulatory medical unit is a unique feature for this hospital that enhances its attractiveness to prospective patients. The teaching-hospital staff is attractive. Having patient information available to set expectations about what will happen through the course of the day is a feature that most patients appreciate. Finally, proactive communication with the family and primary care physician may not have been essential but certainly was desirable. Any unsolicited initiation by clinicians is genuinely appreciated by patients, families, and colleagues.

Other issues related to deficiencies and features can be identified. The bottom line is this: identifying and addressing important deficiencies and features in hospital care is the job of clinician leaders and managers. The following is another hypothetical case example from a managed-care organization.

### Case Example: An Asthmatic Child Needs Medical Attention

The Smith family joined the Happy Healthy HMO (HHH) when Mr. Smith changed employers. It was the first time the family had belonged to a managed-care organization. There are two children in the family, one girl who is healthy, and one boy, age fifteen, who has asthma.

It took nine weeks for the membership materials and identification card to arrive. In the meantime, the boy ran out of his medication and had an acute asthma attack. Since the Smiths had yet to pick a new pediatrician, Mrs. Smith took the wheezing boy to the local hospital emergency room for treatment. He was treated there for sixteen hours and finally improved sufficiently to be treated as an outpatient. There was no place for Mrs. Smith to wait comfortably, so she went to the hospital cafeteria and periodically checked back for a progress report. The boy and his mother were given prescriptions for antibiotics and bronchodilators, with written instructions about things to watch for. They were instructed to follow up with their primary care physician.

#### Continuity of Care

The next day the ER staff called to check on the patient. He had developed a rash. The mother explained that her son has a penicillin allergy, which they had forgotten to mention the day before. The antibiotic was stopped and another prescription was called in to a pharmacy. He was reminded to schedule a follow-up appointment.

The next day, Mrs. Smith made five phone calls before she could locate a physician with HHH that was accepting new patients. This doctor's office was thirty minutes away, and his first available appointment was in two weeks. The boy remained at home from school for four days. Mrs. Smith used up all of her sick time caring for the boy at home. By the time he saw his new doctor, he was wheezing again and had quit the soccer team. Mrs. Smith felt criticized by the doctor for not taking better care of her son. She silently decided to find a new doctor. She called HHH and this time member services was able to guide her to a physician with an interest in asthma whose office was just fifteen minutes from their home.

### Billing and Administration

A month later the Smiths' membership packets arrived. The same week, several bills arrived as well. The ER and pharmacy were not within the HHH network of providers, and the Smiths were expected to pay those bills, even though they have coverage for these services. Mr. Smith registered a complaint about HHH with his benefits manager at work and decided to change insurance with the next open enrollment period. Mr. Smith was called the next day by a member service representative who apologized and waived the bills. Mr. Smith decided to give HHH one more chance but also told the story of the "HMO in disarray" to four friends over lunch.

### Analysis

In this case example, there are deficiencies in care processes as well as features that may or may not foster member loyalty. The delay in distributing membership materials is a common defect among managed-care organizations; it probably contributed to delay in treatment in this case. There were deficiencies in communication around drug allergies and penicillin use. Access to care in a timely manner is assumed in a quality organization. Having to wait two weeks without clinical follow-up may have caused the relapse. Some would argue the physician's interpersonal style that led to the mother feeling judged was suboptimal.

Other examples in this case study are related to features. Offering a service that matches new members with appropriate and accessible primary care physicians may be worth investing in for this HMO. The lack of an attractive waiting room may not compromise care but is certainly undesirable if the emergency room is going to be a welcome place to come to for care. While it is always preferable to prevent errors, the apologetic personal call to Mr. Smith succeeded in recovering his business. Recovery strategies are not essential, but they are features that may help to retain customers.

These case studies highlight the complexity and multidimensional nature of quality. They demonstrate that within the daily work of patient care, there are many examples of deficiencies and features. Optimizing care by measuring and reducing important deficiencies is crucial. It needs to be combined with a careful strategy for enhancing features that attract and retain patients.

## Judging Quality

Another way to look at quality is to recognize that it is judged in two ways:

Quality in fact—objective measures of specific care processes and their outcomes

Quality in perception—subjective evaluations of quality, outcome, and service

### Quality in Fact

Thanks to the efforts of quality assurance professionals and health services researchers, the methods for measuring quality improve every year (Goldfield, Pine, and Pine, 1991; Joint Commission,

1993b). While tremendous methodologic challenges exist, significant progress has been made in the effort to find valid and reliable measures of quality, performance, cost, outcomes, and satisfaction (Siu and others, 1992). Increasingly, purchasers expect quantitative documentation or indicators of hospital and HMO quality (Goldfield and Nash, 1989; Jennison Goonan, 1992; Roper, Winkenwerder, Hackbarth, and Krakauer, 1988). Examples include complication rates, procedure appropriateness rates, and severity-adjusted clinical outcome rates (Joint Commission, 1990). Survey methodologies have evolved and can be considered another objective source of reporting on certain patient-care experiences.

In the past, the patient was viewed as a source of perceptual but not factual information about health care experiences. Recent research disputes this limited role of patient surveys (Greenfield and others, 1988; Kaplan and Ware, 1989; Nelson and Batalden, 1993).

## Quality in Perception

Until fairly recently, health care was judged on reputation and anecdote. In the absence of factual performance information, patients and purchasers naturally relied solely on expert opinion and personal reference. Over the past decade, significant progress has been made in the measurement of perception. Valid and reliable tools exist to monitor the patient's perceptions of care. Extensive research has shown patient perceptions of quality as well as satisfaction with care are essential in the assessment of health care. Perceptions clearly play a major role in physician, hospital, and health plan selection.

## The Balance of Quality Measures

Evaluating quality requires measuring both quality in fact and quality in perception (Townsend with Gebhart, 1990; see Figure 2.1). To focus only on quality in perception is risky. Every hospital and HMO will soon be expected to report on objective performance measures to their purchasers, if not to the public. Without objective

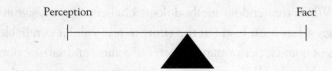

Figure 2.1.  The Quality Balance.

performance information in addition to favorable perceptions of quality, an unusual case of rare but dramatically poor quality can severely tarnish that perception. Similarly, even an organization with outstanding objective performance needs to listen to the patients' perceptions and attend to the concerns they identify. World-class outcomes will not lead to high patient volumes if people perceive the physicians as substandard or the staff as uncaring. Eventually, focusing on one aspect to the neglect of the other will lead to an unsuccessful practice or hospital in most cases.

The problem with measurements of both quality in fact and quality in perception is the lack of practical tools. There continues to be a tremendous need to span the distance between research tools and day-to-day management of a group practice, managed-care organization, or hospital. This dearth of actionable tools and techniques for clinical leaders and managers is one of several driving forces for vertical and horizontal integration of health care organizations. To address the measurement of quality adequately requires a significant capacity for operational research and measurement. Using even existing measurement tools for complication rates, appropriateness of care, quality indicators, outcomes, and patient surveys requires in-house or contracted research expertise. This issue will be explored further in later chapters.

It is important to note that perception is usually measured by patient reports through surveys, interviews, focus groups, and so on. Facts about care can also be measured through patient reports; surveys can determine both factual quality and perceptual quality. For example, patients can be an accurate source of information about what procedures they have had or whether they understand how to take their medications. Other sources for factual measurement are the medical record and administrative data bases.

Examples of specific measures for quality in both perception and fact follow.

*Perception Measures*

Telephone interview data from patients report that they are dissatisfied with your hospital emergency room triage and admitting process.

Survey data from families of patients indicate that they are very satisfied with your HMO's ability to treat chronic depression.

Focus groups of postsurgical patients report the floor nurses do not seem attentive to sanitation, making them question the safety of the institution as a whole.

Patient surveys indicate low confidence in mental health providers in an HMO's network.

*Factual Measures*

Patients treated at your hospital for asthma have higher rates of readmission within thirty days than those treated at competitor hospitals.

Patients in your HMO return to work after myocardial infarction significantly sooner than those being treated by other HMOs (adjusted for severity of illness).

At least 90 percent of myocardial infarction patients in your HMO have follow-up visits scheduled within two weeks of hospital discharge.

## The Process Approach

All work, including clinical practice, is accomplished through processes. Processes are sequentially related steps intended to produce specific outcomes. When a process functions optimally, there is a minimum of wasted effort necessary to achieve the desired outcomes. The process approach is central to all other quality management concepts and methodologies. It provides a concrete framework within which to evaluate, design, and improve clinical practice patterns and patient-care results.

A process has five basic elements (see Figure 2.2):

1. Inputs: in health care, the inputs are patients with their diagnoses and comorbidities.

2. A sequence of steps: a care process or pathway used to prevent, diagnose, or treat illness.

3. Outputs: the process results in terms of patient status, satisfaction, and total cost of services.

4. Suppliers: people and institutions that provide care.

5. Customers: patients, families, purchasers, and others with an interest in the results.

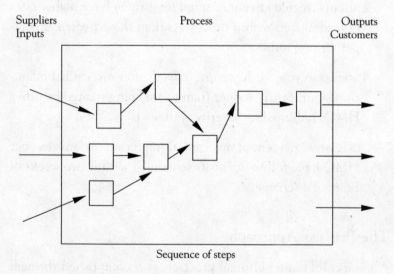

Figure 2.2. The Process Approach.

In clinical care, patients, specimens, information, and other inputs move through processes that change them. This framework provides a taxonomy for discussing and analyzing the value of our clinical practice patterns. Applying process tools in daily work enables clinicians to identify best practices and communicate them among staff and colleagues through protocols, pathways, and guidelines. The process approach allows clinicians to negotiate and clarify everyone's responsibilities in caring for patients.

The degree to which health care services achieve desired health outcomes is determined by four types of factors:

1. A patient's own disease process and severity (inputs)
2. The appropriateness and efficacy of the process of care (process)
3. Patient compliance (process)
4. Random or unidentifiable factors

For the purpose of continuous improvement, it is crucial to know how and where practitioners have control over the results of care. The diagnosis and disease severity must be accounted for when measuring process variation and outcomes, making comparisons, and drawing conclusions about quality of care. Process of care factors pertain to health care providers' capacity to provide optimal care and increase the probability of desired health outcomes. Patient compliance is a matter of debate. Current trends in report cards hold providers and health plans accountable for patient compliance. Random factors are those that cannot be controlled by provider or patient but influence the level of patient results nonetheless. Quality improvement activities need to focus on factors that can be controlled by providers.

### Relevance for Clinicians

In today's environment of competition and accountability, health care organizations are expected to justify how they care for patients and why their approach is cost-effective relative to other peer organizations. To succeed, organizations need a method for describing, judging, and improving care processes and their outcomes.

In many respects, the process approach is akin to applied epidemiology because both approaches group similar patients for the purpose of analyzing their risks, care, and outcomes. Both assume that patients can be grouped into cohorts of comparable individuals. Both strive to compare process and outcomes of their care. Most important, both require full disclosure of the limitations of any conclusions or findings. Rather than fitting clinical practice into a manufacturing mentality, TQM is actually a methodologic cousin to epidemiology and traditional scientific method.

### Use in Improving Clinical Practice

The process approach is a simple yet elegant way to understand clinical practice and to evaluate how well we achieve our intentions. The critical element that allows the application of process improvement theory to patient care is really an epidemiologic concept—stratification. Patients can be stratified into cohorts of comparable patients. Cohort formation should result in groupings of patients that are comparable as "process inputs," that can be reasonably expected to receive comparable diagnostics and treatments, and for which the outcomes of treatment are comparable. If we are to understand and evaluate the quality of care delivered to women with breast cancer, only cohorts of patients with comparable disease risk, type, stage, severity, and comorbidity can be analyzed for their process and outcomes of care.

Processes are the focus of quality management projects. Clinicians drive many processes where the patient is the customer either directly or indirectly, but most processes also involve other personnel, family members, managed-care organizations, and other factors beyond the control of clinicians. The patient plays a major role in every clinical process. The more complex a process is, the harder it is to manage its quality. This is particularly true in clinical care, where patients' needs vary widely and the science of evaluating care is underdeveloped. Because health care processes are highly complex and diverse, there is added opportunity for deficiencies.

The process approach is the basis for a number of clinical decision-making tools such as care paths (see Exhibit 2.1), guidelines, and algorithms (see Figure 2.3). The use of these tools is discussed in later chapters.

### Process Deficiencies

There are two types of defects: errors of execution and errors in handoff. Misreading an ECG or incorrectly sterilizing a surgical field is an error of execution. When an individual improperly executes a task, whether it is a surgical procedure or a medical record notation, there may be consequences for overall patient care, cost, and others involved in caring for the patient.

Exhibit 2.1.  Sample Care Path.

| Day<br>Activities | Pre-Op | Op day | Post-Op<br>day 1 | Post-Op<br>day 2 |
|---|---|---|---|---|
| Tests | ☐ Weight<br>☐ CBC, PT, PTT<br>☐ Type and cross<br>☐ EKG | ☐ Oxygen<br>☐ I's & O's | ☐ Culture drainage | ☐ None |
| Treatments | ☐ IV | ☐ Anesthesia<br>☐ Pain control<br>☐ Fluids | ☐ Wound care<br>☐ Pain control<br>☐ Fluids | ☐ Wound care<br>☐ Pain control<br>☐ Heplock IV |
| Activity | ☐ Education<br>☐ As tolerated | Bed rest | ☐ Review pathway<br>☐ Dangle<br>☐ Diet as tolerated | Up in room |
| Outcomes | ☐ Patient prepared<br>☐ Pre-Op on chart | ☐ Fluid balance<br>☐ Pain control | ☐ Fluid balance<br>☐ Pain control | ☐ Begin activity<br>☐ Drain removal<br>☐ Temp < 100 |

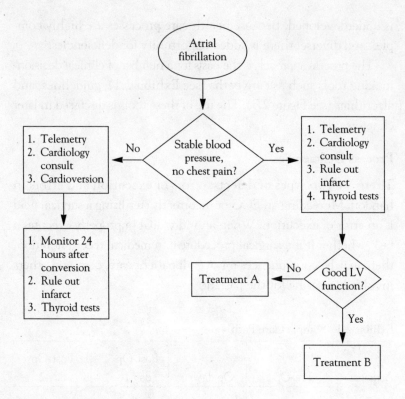

Figure 2.3.  Sample Algorithm.

Errors in handoffs occur when specific tasks within a care process are performed correctly but the handoff between suppliers is defective. Process deficiencies resulting from handoff problems are common; for example, when an abnormal lab test never gets to the ordering physician or when a specialist makes the correct assessment but the assessment fails to reach the primary care physician in a timely manner.

## Customer Focus

Customer focus is one of the fundamental principles of TQM. Not surprisingly, the concept seems almost abhorrent to many clinicians when they think about patients. Similarly, it seems improper to think about the interests of payers and purchasers simultaneously while caring for patients. The word *customer* connotes a commercial relationship, one that has no place in caring for patients.

TQM jargon is not always helpful, particularly if it fosters resistance among clinical professionals. However, the *concept* of customer is applicable to any endeavor. As applied to patient care, it can be helpful to clinicians. The following three illustrations exemplify how the concept applies to current challenges facing health care professionals.

## Case Example: Physician as Customer

An independent practice association called LMD-IPA is experiencing serious financial difficulties. LMD-IPA was started by independent practitioners in a state where competition with staff-model HMOs is fierce. Now it has five hundred member-providers and must reduce its cost structure and control utilization.

On one particular day, numerous elderly patients call physicians' offices to complain about a change in their Medicare plan. They had received letters canceling their Medicare policies through the IPA. The patients were naturally very upset, and office staff members spent much of the day handling these confusing calls. There was no advance notice of this major administrative change.

Two days later letters arrived at most physicians' offices explaining that because the plan is losing $50 per member per month on Medicare patients, the IPA was terminating its Medicare contract. The letter went on to answer some of the questions patients were likely to ask about this change. Not surprisingly, physicians and their office staffs were furious. They expected to be consulted about this type of policy decision. Receiving notification two days after their patients left them uninformed and embarrassed, adding insult to injury.

In this story, physicians are customers of the IPA communication process and suppliers of information to patients who called with questions. Their needs and interests were neglected. Not surprisingly, physicians and their staff were so angered by the way they were treated that they actively criticized LMD-IPA to their patients. These process deficiencies will likely translate into loss of market share for the IPA.

### Case Example: Patient as Customer

A woman was readmitted to All-purpose Academic Medical Center (AAMC) at 2:00 A.M. in hypoglycemic coma. She had been discharged from AAMC less than twenty-four hours previously, after a fourteen-day stay for new-onset insulin-dependent diabetes. On readmission, the patient arrived by ambulance from a homeless shelter with a blood sugar of 23.

On morning rounds, the resident described the patient's previous admission. She had presented two weeks previously, moderately ketotic and dehydrated, with a blood sugar of 689. She was treated on the internal medicine ward with consultation from endocrinology, diabetic teaching, and social services. The care she received resulted in tight blood sugar control and the patient had been discharged with a fasting blood sugar of 100, long-acting insulin, syringes, and a follow-up appointment with one of the residents. The hospitalization cost $26,000.

After hearing about the previous admission, the attending physician questioned the patient. It was evident that the patient was learning impaired. She had no syringes or insulin and did not know where they were. When asked to describe the previous day's events, she explained that she returned to the shelter midday and did not eat for the rest of the day, because she does not like the food. She could not describe the evening events or how she got back to the hospital. At the end of the interview, she pulled the attending physician aside and asked for help because she could not read the syringes.

This case study highlights a problem common in health care organizations today: practicing "good" medicine according to the current literature may not necessarily meet the needs of individual patients. Ironically, this patient was not on any pathways or protocols that might have led clinicians to treat her like a patient with more resources for self-care. It appeared that the institution was simply focused on tight blood sugar and the evidence supporting reduction in long-term complications. Meanwhile, this patient was at high risk for life-threatening short-term complications of treatment.

Often clinicians assume TQM implies regimenting care to patients and threats to personalized treatment. On the contrary, meeting customer requirements implies an even greater response to individual patient needs and expectations. Does this notion conflict with the concepts of applied epidemiology described earlier? Yes, it can. It points out the fact that managing clinical care and competing on performance are complex. They require the ability to balance both individual and population perspectives in the management of patients.

### Case Example: Purchaser as Customer

Competent Computer Company (CCC) is a large national company that has an account with your HMO. The company is struggling to succeed in the international market place and is laying off thousands of employees to get costs down and improve competitive position.

CCC has made a commitment to working with managed-care organizations as health care suppliers so it can document and improve the value of care it purchases for employees and their dependents. The company has a list of expectations that includes a variety of measurements it expects your management to report on every six months. It expects to see performance measurement and improvement results over time.

The chairman of internal medicine is expected to present progress against improvement goals to CCC on a regular basis. The requirements for internal medicine measurements include physician-specific practice profiling of prevention screening, test ordering, referral use, hospital use, and functional outcome measures for angina and asthma patients. CCC does not expect to see the results on individual physicians, but it does expect to see planwide results and to be informed on performance improvement.

At a recent site visit, the HMO was harshly criticized because it has not demonstrated improvement on its measures. There were threats of terminating the contract. CCC wants to see measurement, but more important, it wants to see improvement against those measures. It expects to see a plan from the internal medicine department that specifies strategic, annual, and tactical goals for improvement. New enrollment in the HMO is closed until performance improvement is documented.

The chairman of internal medicine must face his colleagues and explain this development. He must find a way to communicate the purchaser's expectations so that they are motivated to take these issues seriously and to contribute time to changing practice patterns.

This case study highlights several concerns clinicians have about the concept of customer. A major concern is that physicians assume purchasers are simply interested in price. Many clinicians see purchaser initiatives as thinly veiled attempts to save money. Another concern is that the science of quality measurement is underdeveloped and there is tremendous fear about unfair use of inaccurate information. There is some evidence to suggest that this fear may be justified from markets where purchaser-driven data have been used to expose or exclude capable practitioners. A third problem is practitioners' lack of knowledge about quality measurement and assumptions about the waste of effort these initiatives may engender. Each of these concerns is understandable. All are surmountable through greater awareness, information, and responsible actions and accountability.

## Who Are "Customers"?

"Customer" is only a concept, a way of thinking about all those affected by our work. It means anyone who depends on us for some service or product. It is helpful to think of customers from two perspectives: external and internal.

## External Customers

There are three basic external customer groups for HMOs and hospitals. The first and most obvious is patients. While doctors take their responsibility to individual patients very seriously, issues such as those raised in the "Patient as Customer" case illustrate how practitioners can become focused inward on professional standards at the expense of patients. Customer concepts have been used to redesign care processes to focus on patients' priorities and make clinicians even more effective (Nelson and Wasson, 1993).

A second group of external customers includes payers and purchasers such as insurance companies, employers, or government agencies—the parties who pay the medical bills and select the health plans for patients. Increasingly, they see themselves as educated purchasers, not simply payers.

A third group of external customers includes various regulators such as the Joint Commission on Accreditation of Health Care Organizations, the National Committee on Quality Assurance, state health and data agencies, and so on.

Some health care organizations also consider the community as a whole as a customer group. This vision implies that these organizations consider the overall health status of their community a part of their responsibilities. Physicians can be customers of health care organizations, particularly in relation to administrative functions and processes. Institutions such as nursing homes and acute-care hospitals can be each other's customers. Successful patient transfers require knowing and understanding customer needs for patient status, records, timing, and so on. The external customers of a hospital are displayed in Figure 2.4.

## Internal Customers

Internal customers are those people within your organization who are affected in some way by your work (see Figure 2.5). Satisfying external customers requires that we also satisfy the needs of our internal customers. For LMD-IPA in the case study above, there was a lack of commitment to meeting the needs and expectations of

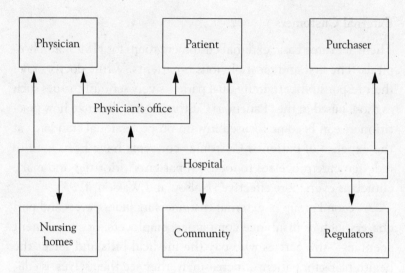

Figure 2.4. External Customers.

internal customers (contracted primary care physicians). The result was confused patients, hostile network physicians, and shrinking market share for the IPA.

In clinical practice, there are many examples of the importance of teamwork between internal customers within a care process. In a major analysis of mortality and other outcomes of cardiac surgery in Pennsylvania, analysis of causes of variation in mortality rates led researchers to conclude that teamwork may have played a role (Williams, Nash, and Goldfield, 1991). On a smaller scale, one of the most common causes of resource waste and patient hazard found by clinical teams relates to handoffs between clinical staff. For example, a number of organizations have reduced the post-operative wound infection rate by improving the timing of prophylactic antibiotic administration. While physicians typically order the drugs, there are often deficiencies due to handoff problems that result in drugs not getting administered properly. Defining internal customers' needs in the drug-prescribing process is a crucial step for projects seeking to reduce the postoperative wound infection rate.

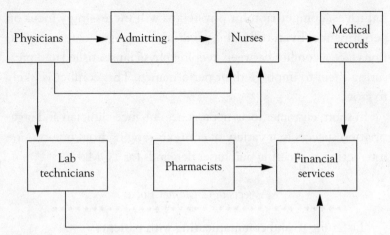

Figure 2.5. Internal Customers.

The terms *customer* and *supplier* can apply to the same individual. Physicians may be internal customers of an internal hospital process as well as suppliers in relation to the patient as the external customers of overall care. These terms provide a language to analyze individual responsibilities as well as needs. They are only concepts. Use them in quality management work only if and when they help clarify roles.

### Why Is Customer Focus Important?

Until the 1970s, there was thought to be a shortage of physicians and hospitals for the demand for access to medical care. Government programs subsidized medical education and institutional growth. While the problem of access and specialty maldistribution continue to plague underserved communities, increasingly health care organizations must compete for patients and purchasers. Meeting customer requirements for features as well as defect-free care is a major challenge. Its importance will grow, as techniques develop to measure customer expectations and ratings of care.

Similarly, hospitals and managed-care organizations must increasingly compete for high-performing clinicians. As the science of quality measurement develops and the capacity to assess practice improves, competition for physicians will increasingly focus on performance. Even today, hospitals and managed-care organizations face a conflict between keeping physicians satisfied and pressuring them to improve their performance. This conflict is likely to grow.

In short, customer focus approaches enhance clinician and organization success in a variety of contexts ranging from one-on-one interaction to meeting purchaser demands for TQM.

*Aspects of Customer Focus*

Listening to and communicating with patients

Optimizing treatment patterns and outcomes

Enhancing the quality and efficiency of internal processes

Designing patient-focused care

Responding to purchaser expectations

## Customer Focus with Individual Patients

Communication skills are not given much emphasis in most medical schools and residency training programs. One place communication skills get some attention is in risk management courses on loss prevention. In this context, physicians are taught that it is important to go beyond providing technically correct care. The lesson usually taught is that patients need to have the opportunity to describe their complaints in full, even when the physician can make the diagnosis with less conversation. Without this opportunity, patients are more likely to complain or consider litigation (Delbanco, 1992; Quill, 1989).

Not only do unhappy patients consider litigation, they change doctors and health plans and often tell their friends and colleagues about their negative experiences. This negative advertising travels widely and lasts a long time in a community. They also do not bond as closely to their physician. There is some evidence to suggest they are not as compliant with treatment recommendations when they have not had the opportunity to tell their story (Eraker, 1984; Smith and Hoppe, 1991).

Fee-for-service practitioners in solo or small group practice find these concepts self-evident. If they do not focus on satisfying patients, their practices will not survive. Physicians salaried by HMOs or managed-care organizations can be insulated from the demands of patients for attentive, personal interrelationships. Few clinicians in any context receive quantitative and qualitative information about their professional style with patients. Not surprisingly, managed-care organizations around the country are starting to experiment with physician-specific patient satisfaction measurement. In some instances, this includes incentive pay based on these measures (Schlackman, 1989).

Practitioners with managed-care contracts find themselves boxed in between patients who fear their incentives to withhold treatment and utilization management programs that discourage resource use. These conflicting incentives and pressures may grow as capitation and global budgeting become more common means of payment. Customer concepts can be helpful in navigating these circumstances.

### Case Example: A Patient with Headaches

Consider a patient who presents complaining of chronic headaches. The patient has had headaches for ten years, they are unchanged, and there are no neurologic symptoms or findings on exam. The patient's uncle has recently been diagnosed with brain cancer. She wants a CT scan. She distrusts the physician's judgment that a CT scan is not indicated because she knows that the physician contracts with an HMO. The physician gets impatient with her for questioning his professional judgment. The patient shops around in the HMO until she finds a doctor who will give her a CT scan. The test result comes back normal.

The headaches continue, along with the patient's anxiety. After reading an article in a lay magazine about magnetic resonance scanning, she returns requesting an MRI scan. She continues to believe that something serious is wrong. After several more tests and visits, she finally comes to realize that her health is intact. To lose weight, she starts a regular exercise program. Weeks later she notes that her headaches appear to have almost resolved.

How can customer concepts help in this case? The clinician's role is to ferret out the true needs and concerns of a patient so that they can be fully met. TQM teaches the importance of systematically identifying and addressing true customer (patient) needs. This patient does not need a CT scan; she needs convincing reassurance that she does not have brain cancer. The key is to identify and address the underlying need, not the superficial expressed need for a test. In this case, the physician became defensive about his clinical judgment, and his defensiveness may have fueled the patient's apprehensions. A more effective strategy would be to explore the stated need to uncover the true need, the need that must be met to satisfy the customer's requirements. Sometimes an unnecessary test is unavoidable. In many cases, effective reassurance combined with information and compassion will meet the patient's true need. It will also build trust, respect, and loyalty in the relationship. Enhanced communication skills can improve a practitioner's success in these cases.

One way to explore this directly is to use a simple survey in daily practice. Some clinicians have their office staff hand out surveys one day or half day a week for a few weeks every six months. This provides a fairly random sample of patient evaluations at periodic intervals. The feedback can be surprising and educational.

The questions can be very simple:

What did you like about this visit?

What did you dislike about this visit?

Do you have any other feedback you would like to give the
doctor or staff?

On a scale of 1 to 5, how would you rate the visit?

The five-point scale in the last question can be converted into
percentage of satisfied patients by using the following formula:

$$\frac{\text{Total of all scores}}{\text{Number of patients seen}} \times 20 = \text{percent satisfied}$$

This percentage can be plotted on a graph and tracked over time
(see Figure 2.6). This type of simple but informative measurement
can provide clinicians with immediate feedback about their personal style with patients. As the figure implies, a common result of
such personal feedback is that interpersonal style improves and

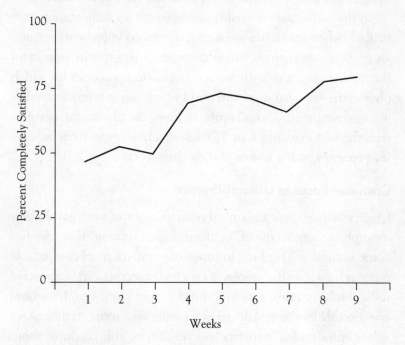

Figure 2.6. Run Chart, Patient Satisfaction.

patient satisfaction increases. Obviously, this simple measurement would not meet the rigorous standards required for external reporting, judgment, or comparison. It is simply designed for personal use and improvement.

## Customer Focus with Colleagues and Staff

In addition to the value of customer concepts in dealings with patients, another critical application is in internal care processes. There are a myriad of complex processes that "produce" health care, processes that are often invisible to the patient.

Often it is the internal processes, such as distributing lab results or administering drugs, that are major sources of waste and hazard to patients. The outputs of internal processes are essential to high-quality, efficient care. Practitioners are often the customers of internal processes because they depend on so many institutional functions to complete diagnostic and therapeutic steps in patient care.

In the early stages of quality management implementation, particularly when physicians are skeptical, starting improvement teams for processes with physicians as customers helps to win support for the quality program. Early success improving processes for which physicians are customers can build physician interest in quality management methods and projects. From the physicians' perspective, the best evidence that TQM is effective comes from improving processes highly visible in their daily work.

## Customer Focus in Clinical Practice

Quality management in clinical practice requires a mental shift for most physicians, a type of "epidemiologic thinking" that may not come naturally. Thinking in terms of populations of comparable patients for whom the process of care and outcomes can be expected to be similar requires a mental shift for most clinicians. It requires considerable intellectual dexterity to maintain a focus on the unique needs of individual patients and yet also be able to think about whole populations. Clinician managers should be aware of this.

Once clinicians accept this way of thinking scientifically about their patients as groups or cohorts, the door is open to clinical quality management. Until they see the value of viewing their practices in this manner, it is common to experience explicit and implicit resistance to measurement and improvement of clinical processes.

### Customer Focus with Purchasers and Payers

Many clinicians are beginning to feel the pressure of market-area competition. Typically, however, it is only physician managers who actually come face to face with representatives from purchasers assessing the quality and efficiency of hospitals and HMOs.

Exposing the front-line clinicians to the needs and expectations of purchasers can be extremely valuable. Health care purchasers and their consultants are far more sophisticated today than in the past. It is inaccurate to assume their concerns are limited to cost. Often, they are open and eager to collaborate on quality measurement and management initiatives. They can be very helpful to medical managers who find themselves browbeating colleagues into participating in the quality program. Purchasers create more positive and realistic motivation for physicians than the traditional regulatory mentality sometimes associated with quality assurance. Many physicians recognize the legitimate concerns of corporate America about the value of health care they purchase.

In some cases, economic survival drives an openness to the needs and expectations of purchasers. In other situations, the appeal is more intellectual, based on an awareness of the American health care financing crisis. Regardless, creating opportunities for clinicians to interact with external customers about their expectations can help build support for a clinical quality management program.

Table 2.2 is an example of purchaser expectations about clinical quality and performance measurement. It displays the request of the primary customer (the purchaser) for information about quality and cost. While this is the primary need, more detailed secondary needs clarify what information the hospital or health plan

Table 2.2. Purchaser Expectations.

| Primary Need | Secondary Need | Supplier Translation | Measure |
|---|---|---|---|
| Assessment of quality and efficiency | Outcomes | Functional status | Measure of 3 diagnoses |
| | Cost per case | Case management cost savings | Time trend savings |
| | Defect rates | Surgical complications | Complication rates versus benchmarks |
| | Cost per diagnosis | Length of stay by diagnosis group | Time trend Length of stay |

must provide. These secondary needs can be translated into topics the supplier (hospital or HMO) needs to address. Finally, measures can then be assigned to the quality department for further specification, data collection, analysis, and reporting.

## Variation

Analysis of variation in clinical practice is fundamental to quality management. Variation in clinical practice is often defended as the art of medicine or professional autonomy. But unintended variation—that is, variation in practice patterns without a clear purpose in caring for patients—is a major source of unnecessary waste and potential hazard (Berwick, 1991). Today, patients and purchasers want assurance that outcomes, practice patterns, and resource use comply with proven norms for cost-effective health care. Increasingly, corporate leaders voice awareness of the challenges clinicians face in meeting this expectation, but they have grown impatient with medicine's rate of response and lack of success. Health care organizations are expected to overcome the obstacles to valid measurement and demonstrate an ability to manage variation appropriately.

All processes vary; no process functions exactly the same over time. Some variation is desirable, such as that intended to meet the unique needs of unique patients. Often, however, variation is undesirable. Unintended variation wastes resources and leads to variation in outcomes. It can lead to poor quality. It often costs more but does not add to the quality of care. Reducing unintended or inappropriate variation is a fundamental aspect of clinical quality management.

What do we mean by practice variation? Here are two examples. Some physicians are skeptical about using aspirin in unstable angina patients because they are afraid of bleeding complications, despite the overwhelming scientific evidence that it is generally safe and effective at reducing future cardiac events. Analyses of their practices reveal that severity-adjusted rates of recurrent myocardial infarctions are more frequent among their patients (Willard, Lange, and Hillis, 1992).

Consider a second example of unintended and undesirable variation. The lab at a certain hospital has not specified a consistent process for managing stat pregnancy tests. At night, the processing takes hours longer than during the day because the technicians use a different process. The rate of missed ectopic and ruptured ectopic pregnancy is higher at night than during the day.

In both examples, characteristics of a particular care process demonstrate trends that warrant further inquiry. These trends strongly suggest patterns in practice that vary from the scientific evidence or intention. In both examples, some corrective action is necessary.

## Two Types of Variation

Process variation can be classified into two types. According to the scientist who developed this concept, Walter Shewhart ([1939] 1986), variation in processes and outcomes must be understood if we are to manage processes and achieve predictable, optimal results. For clinical leaders, the distinction is important. Different management approaches are successful with each type of variation.

Random variation (also known as common cause variation) is variation that is intrinsic to the process design. Random variation in response to a particular treatment occurs even among cohorts of comparable patients. For example, for a cohort of patients with uncomplicated essential hypertension, there will always be some variation in the response to a treatment plan of beta blockers and diuretics. Even for one individual patient, there will be variability in response over time. There is, however, an overall predictable level of response to particular drug regimens within a cohort of comparable patients.

Assignable variation (also known as special cause variation) is extrinsic to the usual process, related to identifiable patient or physiologic characteristics, unusual or idiosyncratic practice patterns, and other identifiable process characteristics. Assignable variation can be traced to root cause and managed without changing the underlying care process. The care process may be the right process, but assignable causes of variation require attention.

Consider the following examples. Although individual practitioners manage uncomplicated essential hypertension somewhat differently, there is a general process of care based on current professional knowledge, community standards, and perhaps a clinical guideline. Differences in frequency of visits or lab tests, number of weeks to return to normotension, and side effect rates will exist; some variation is random and intrinsic to the care process. Variable physiologic response, level of patient compliance, frequency of dose (or dosing) adjustments, and unknown factors create random variation. It is reasonable, however, to expect blood pressure reduction on standard treatment plans, within a predictable range of response. Lack of response raises questions about the accuracy of the diagnosis, patient noncompliance, and other possible assignable causes.

While practitioners can expect a certain level of response to usual treatment for essential hypertension, there may be a subset of patients who develop intolerable side effects from the medication and refuse treatment. The cause of the poor response to the treatment plan is assignable. In addition, the annual cost of achieving blood pressure control can vary in assignable ways. On average, the annual cost of managing essential uncomplicated hypertension can be measured and a range of random variation defined. However, some practitioners may believe that patients should be seen more often or have more blood chemistry tests than their colleagues do. The patients of these practitioners will have higher annual costs than comparable hypertension patients. There may be a subset of patients who do not take diuretics regularly because they are embarrassed by frequent urination. If they are also too self-conscious to make this problem known to their physician, one might conclude that they are responding to the drug poorly. Each of these exemplifies assignable variation.

The mathematical rules of probability and prediction often apply in patient care. However, assignable causes of variation make mathematical prediction about process performance and the probability of outcomes impossible. Identifying and minimizing all assignable cause of variation is a prerequisite to defining the effectiveness of a diagnostic or treatment plan.

The difficulties arise from the paucity of scientifically derived evidence about which practices are causally related to desired outcomes (Eddy, 1990a, 1990b). The question of professional uncertainty is an issue of major debate and research. Management of processes to optimize their efficiency and quality requires understanding their variability. Wherever possible, assignable and random variation must be identified. Assignable causes should be addressed and reduced; then the process and its effectiveness can be determined, the ultimate goal being improved outcomes for whole cohorts and populations.

Because random and assignable variation are different, each requires a different management response:

- Random variation: new performance is achieved by process redesign and innovation; no focused case review is needed.

- Assignable variation: case-by-case focused review is warranted to identify causes and take appropriate action.

Quality management professionals have developed extensive statistical and analytical techniques to facilitate interpretation of variation (Juran, 1988).

### Process Capability

After assignable variation in a care process has been traced to assignable causes and reduced, the care process can be evaluated for its capacity to achieve desired outcomes. As Walter Shewhart would say, the process capability can be measured. Process capability refers to the measurable rates of negative events (deficiencies such as preventable complications) or positive events (desired outcomes such as early return to function after hip fracture). For key clinical processes, capability is the measure of success in achieving optimal results and minimal cost.

## The Health Care Research Spectrum

Medical education and the historic basic research focus on the discovery of new interventions have skewed the medical profession's perspective on the role of research. In engineering for other professions and industries, there is a commonly accepted role for research across a spectrum of applications, from basic science to operations. This spectrum allows us to apply to health care an important general concept developed by Genichi Taguchi, a Japanese engineer and innovator of research methodologies and applications (Ross, 1988). It helps to clarify the role of measurement, planning, and improvement in clinical practice. Taguchi defined the distinction between off-line and on-line research (see Figure 2.7). Off-line research represents the design functions conducted in experimental settings; on-line research involves assessing whether practice patterns proven to produce optimal outcomes are in use (Jennison Goonan and Jordan, 1992).

At the far left end of off-line research is the study of raw materials or inputs into processes. For health care, this is the work of

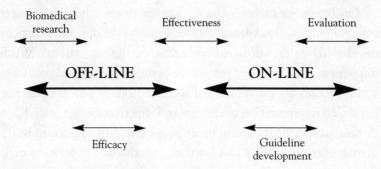

Figure 2.7.  Health Care Research Continuum.
*Source:* © *Quality Review Bulletin* 18(11). Oakbrook Terrace, IL: Joint Commission on Accreditation of Healthcare Organizations, 1992, pp. 372–379. Reprinted with permission.

biomedical research to understand human physiology and disease pathology. It is a prerequisite to designing medical interventions that achieve optimal outcomes.

After the study of our inputs comes efficacy research, which identifies, in highly controlled settings, diagnostic and therapeutic interventions that have the desired impact on patients. Efficacy research builds from the knowledge of biomedical research and attempts to design diagnostic tests and treatments that are efficacious and safe. The gold-standard design of efficacy research is the randomized controlled trial used to determine causality between treatment and outcome for a population of patients with the comparable diagnoses and risk.

Effectiveness research extends toward the on-line end of the research spectrum. One of its objectives is to identify whether efficacious diagnostic and therapeutic interventions are effective in routine, uncontrolled clinical practice. Effectiveness research provides information about the effectiveness of different intervention strategies, practice patterns, and delivery systems—the information prerequisite to identifying best clinical practice and methods for achieving optimal outcomes. Ideally, it answers the basic questions about what constitutes quality health care and identifies valid measures of process and outcome.

On-line work includes the translation of effectiveness research into guidelines. Guidelines are specifications of optimal practices, developed by practitioners involved in caring for patients. While differences exist, practice parameters, guidelines, critical pathways, and protocols are all variants of specifications of process based on consensus interpretation of efficacy and effectiveness research. Specifications of optimal clinical practice are critically important to the management of quality and lay the groundwork for decision making about what and how to evaluate quality.

At the far end of on-line activities is operational measurement or evaluation. Its purpose is to report continuously on actual performance. Health care organizations' capability to produce such routine quality information is notably underdeveloped. On-line measurement is akin to the work of quality assurance programs but goes beyond regulation-driven reporting to incorporate measures that inform quality improvement activities of a professional group, hospital, or other health care organization. The on-line end of the spectrum is fundamental to quality management processes in clinical practice.

## The Scientific Method and Total Quality Management

TQM is the scientific method applied to the way we manage cohorts of patients within hospitals and health maintenance organizations (see Figure 2.8). It is a practical applied science that cuts through the complexity of academic research and focuses on fixing the myriad problems and deficiencies that get in the way of efficient clinical care. For this reason, many physicians find it applies very naturally to their clinical practice.

When Joseph Juran developed his model for project-by-project quality improvement, he described undertaking a two-phase approach to problem solving: a diagnostic phase and a remedial phase—akin to fundamental clinical decision making. His approach for solving organizational problems relies on the principles of scientific

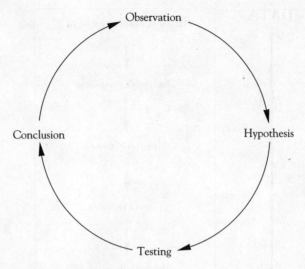

Figure 2.8. Scientific Method.

experimentation (Figure 2.9). Diagnosing process deficiencies requires collecting data on the problem and identifying its root cause. It requires using common sense to identify process changes that will improve quality and efficiency. It does not require running clinical trials at every hospital or HMO, but it does mean collecting actionable information about process and outcomes of care.

Effective problem solving requires applied experimentation to identify solutions that work. While these methods are well understood by most clinicians, they have not been incorporated into the way we function as organizations. We have typically relegated scientific evaluation of what does and does not work to academia, leaving a void on the operational side where applied science is lacking in most institutions.

## Total Quality Management: The Basic Approach

So what does TQM entail? Three basic strategies form the foundation of a quality management program; together they are known as the Juran Trilogy.

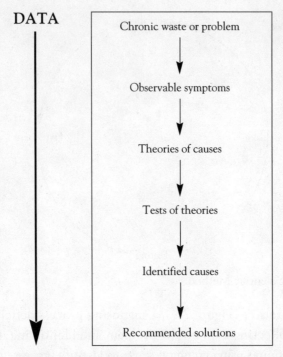

Figure 2.9.  Scientific Method Applied to Process Improvement.

1. *Quality control* includes the activities directed at measuring the quality and efficiency of processes. It involves measuring process and outcomes variables and determining the degree to which they vary from intention. Quality control entails using pathways, practice pattern feedback, and incentives to reduce assignable variation that is undesirable, unnecessary, and inappropriate. In health care it is a set of techniques used to reduce assignable causes of variation in clinical processes so that operational on-line experiments can be used to identify more effective diagnosis and treatment processes. Quality control activities result in more stable and predictable care processes. They are a prerequisite to on-line quality improvement projects to increase process capability.

2. *Quality planning* encompasses the tools and techniques used to design processes that work optimally. In health care, planning techniques are used to develop clinical guidelines and pathways that

are simply specifications of processes. Clinical protocols used in research and clinical trials are also specifications of a process. Any process, from lab result distribution to appointment scheduling to clinical decision making about whether to perform a cardiac catheterization, can be designed to function better using quality planning techniques.

3. *Quality improvement* is a set of tools and methods that can be used once undesirable assignable variation has been eliminated. It entails diagnosing root causes of process performance, conducting on-line experiments to identify more cost-efficient and effective practice patterns, and defining organizational interventions such as training and decision support to adopt new practices and achieve better outcomes.

Together, these three approaches offer a more systematic and comprehensive approach to health care quality and efficiency than anything attempted previously. One crucial skill for quality management professionals to acquire is the ability to judge which approach and which tools are appropriate for solving a specific problem. Many organizations that have implemented continuous improvement programs over the past several years have invested huge resources for relatively limited gain. This is largely because learning how, where, and when to use tools and techniques is a sophisticated skill. It is akin to developing the expertise to know how to manage an intraoperative myocardial infarction or prevent protracted convalescence in an elderly hip fracture patient. These are not simple skills that can be learned from a book. Selection of approach and tools is a skill set worthy of respect. Every organization needs a core of subspecialists with this expertise.

## Accreditation

Accreditation is changing in ways that mirror changes in the industry as a whole. There are two major accreditation programs in

managed care, including the National Committee on Quality
Assurance (1994) and the Joint Commission on Accreditation of
Healthcare Organizations (1993a). Both these accreditation programs have incorporated many of the concepts and principles of
continuous improvement into their standards.

The Joint Commission on Accreditation of Healthcare Organizations (JCAHO) is promoting a related framework for thinking
about quality improvement that it calls performance-based quality-
of-care evaluation. It identifies performance-based evaluation as a
relatively new approach to measuring and improving quality. The
approach, which is fundamental to the 1994 hospital and network
accreditation standards, incorporates the concepts of identifying
variation around intended performance, reducing when appropriate, and improving overall performance of processes of care.

JCAHO identifies three tools to monitor and identify opportunities for improvement (see Figure 2.10): indicators, guidelines and
standards, and a performance data base. An *indicator* is a measure
used to monitor and improve the quality of important governance,
management, clinical, and support services that strongly affect
patient outcomes. A *guideline* is a standardized specification for care
developed by a formal process that incorporates the best scientific
evidence with expert opinion. A *standard* is a statement of expectation that defines an organization's governance, management,

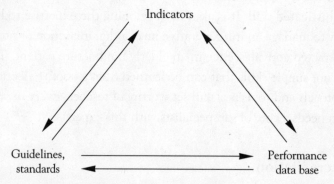

Figure 2.10. Performance-Based Quality Systems.

clinical, and support services capacity to provide quality care. And a *performance data base* is an organized comprehensive collection of data used to produce information relating to the quality of patient care.

## Conclusion

Basic concepts, like basic physiology, only prepare the clinician leader for the skills of the profession. It is a knowledge foundation of terms, definitions, and facts that are useful only if applied to real-life problems. The chapters that follow move from abstract concepts to practical applications.

# 3

. . . . . . . . . . . . . . . . . . . . . . . . . . . . . .

# A Sampler of
# Success Stories

Until about 1990, applications of TQM in clinical practice were rare. There were few published case examples. One had to search to find examples of the use of TQM principles and techniques in clinical practice. Increasingly, TQM is viewed as an application of the scientific method and epidemiological thinking to the care of cohorts of patients. Case studies of successful applications are told at conferences and published in professional journals.

This chapter describes eight stories of TQM projects in clinical care in varied settings with diverse purposes. Each story was selected because it exemplifies the current state of TQM applications in clinical practice. The purpose is to describe cutting-edge success stories of clinical TQM applications in 1994, knowing that this is a field in rapid evolution. Examples from individual institutions were chosen specifically because they represent projects that *any* hospital or group practice could replicate. The goal here is not to critique but rather to identify the accomplishments and opportunities for further development within the field of clinical quality improvement as a whole. Compendiums of case studies exist that provide further case examples (Vibbert, Migdail, Strickland, and Youngs, 1994).

## Postoperative Open-Heart Surgery Care:
## Medical Center Hospital of Vermont (MCHV)

This project is a wonderful example of what a project team can accomplish in a hospital setting. *USA Today* gave it a quality award in 1994. The project objective was explicit: to reduce length of stay while maintaining or improving quality (Schriefer, 1993, p. 8). It was chartered in response to customer (purchaser) demand for reduced cost and length of stay (LOS) for open-heart surgery patients, which were higher at MCHV than at other hospitals in its market area.

Over time, team members grew to see the project as their own, not just a purchaser requirement. As care process deficiencies surfaced, team members developed a sense of ownership and pride that motivated their work. When they initially analyzed the care given to open-heart surgery patients, they realized that there were a number of chronic problems:

- The Surgical Intensive Care Unit (SICU) often filled to capacity, requiring surgeons to postpone cases. This caused patients unnecessary anxiety.

- Many employees believed that practices at MCHV were outdated in certain minor respects that could be causing longer LOS.

- Existing data showed that the average LOS at MCHV was longer than at other comparable hospitals.

A cross-functional team from surgery, anesthesia, recovery room, respiratory therapy, and nursing described the current process using flow charting (Figure 3.1). They collected simple data on current practice patterns regarding drug usage, time intervals for key steps such as intubation, and complications. They tested theories of causes of prolonged intubation by simple data collection and analysis (Figure 3.2). They interviewed patients about

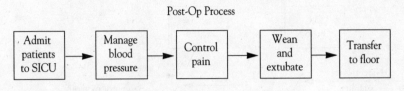

- Flow charting resulting in communication
- Simple process measures
- Causes of narcotic use identified
- Benchmarking with other hospitals

Figure 3.1.  Flow Chart of Current Process.
*Source:* Fletcher Allen Health Care.

their experiences around surgery. With all this information, along with evidence from the medical literature, they developed a "best practice" care pathway and decision algorithms for steps that consistently caused variation.

Following the path was optional, with the understanding that the path would change over time as practitioners found deficiencies in the path itself. Significant effort went into communication about the project and the path through group meetings and educational videotapes. Simple data about practice patterns were collected on a regular basis and fed back to individual practitioners, allowing them to address their own unintended variation. With frequent feedback on a short list of process measures and patient outcomes, clinicians increasingly put their patients on the protocol. Assignable variation was reduced. Today, the majority of patients are on the pathway, and clinicians can focus on other problems.

Another characteristic of the project typical of successful TQM applications was the interdisciplinary teamwork. The team used a highly participatory approach with early recruitment of skeptics and supporters alike. The team overcame the cycle of fear (see Figure 3.3). This cycle illustrates what typically happens when managers attempt to impose changes through top-down approaches. People will criticize the messenger rather than learn from the message. They make efforts to discredit the information or source. As a last

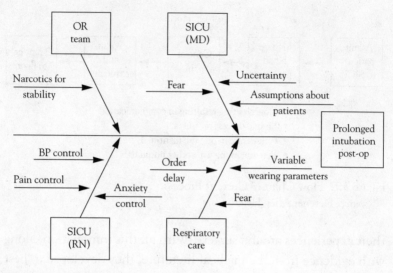

Figure 3.2.  Cause-and-Effect Diagram.
*Source:* Fletcher Allen Health Care.

resort, they will micromanage to camouflage process deficiencies, despite the fact that they may be causing hazard to patients and inefficiencies in patient care. All in all, these defensive maneuvers lead to an atmosphere of fear, defensiveness, and stagnation.

The results of the project are striking. Hours of intubation dropped from an average of 37.2 to 28.7. Total length of stay fell from 12.4 to 10.6 days. Mortality fell to 1.6 percent and reintubation is down to 1.1 percent. These successes have made MCHV a national benchmark.

However, like most process improvement projects, this one did not identify any major innovations in medical practice. Safe techniques of early extubation following cardiac surgery were discovered decades ago (Klineberg, Geer, Hirsh, and Aukburg, 1977; Quasha and others, 1989; Ramsay and others, 1985). The scientific evidence supporting the new practice patterns adopted by MCHV already existed. The team's breakthrough was to discover a way to incorporate current scientific knowledge into routine care for patients.

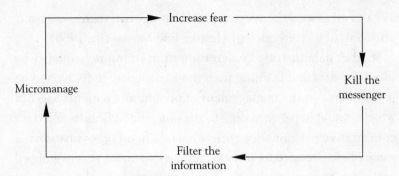

Figure 3.3. The Cycle of Fear.

The team successfully implemented existing efficacy and effectiveness knowledge into routine practice, a very important application of quality management techniques. By doing so, they reduced
unintended and wasteful variability. TQM methods are invaluable
in activities intended to reduce practitioner variability around routine care processes. This project set the stage for innovations in
quality and cost in the open-heart surgery process. Wasteful complexity and variation only obscure the ability to evaluate and
improve care processes.

There is no definitive explanation for the reduction in complication rates in this project. There was no specific intervention
intended to reduce reintubation and mortality rates; it may well be
a form of the Hawthorne effect, a change that occurs coincidentally
but not by design. Ongoing measurement and feedback and general
attentiveness to the process protocol reduced length of stay but also
coincidentally led to improved outcomes.

## Hospital Pneumonia Management:
## Forbes Health System

Forbes was an early user of the MedisGroups system of severity
adjustment and mortality measurement (McGarvey and Harper,

1993). Forbes used the system in its infancy, when there were many criticisms of its methodology (Iezzoni and Moskowitz, 1988).

Forbes demonstrated a determination to improve quality by using the data and learning from the experience. It discovered its performance in the management of pneumonia patients was not what it would hope, according to the outcome indicators and their comparative performance with others. When Forbes first started using MedisGroups data in 1987, the measurement system grouped patients into four severity groups and compared actual to expected rates of major morbidity and mortality for individual hospitals. The number of patients with major morbidity and mortality within the sickest group of patients was higher than expected.

Forbes leaders chartered an interdisciplinary quality improvement team. First, team members brainstormed all possible explanations of their performance level. Then they conducted an exploratory analysis of their existing data to test these hypotheses of causes of their performance. Using their data, they excluded many possible explanations, such as individual physicians with poor practice habits, poor data quality, random variation, and the MedisGroups model itself. The most common explanations were delayed administration of antibiotics and inappropriate choice of drugs or use of subspecialty consultants.

Next the team reviewed a sample of medical records to discover possible causes of delayed administration of antibiotics and inappropriate choice of antibiotic coverage. They also evaluated the use of subspecialists and the timing of cultures. They used a quasi-experimental case-control approach by comparing the care to two groups of matched pneumonia patients. "Cases" were those patients who died and "controls" were patients who lived. A number of potential improvements in several processes were identified. The team found significant variation in timing of sputum culture collection, blood culture collection, timing of antibiotic administration, antibiotic coverage for Legionella and mycoplasma, and the indications for infectious disease and pulmonary consultation.

This diagnostic phase of the project led to redesigning the emergency room process to ensure that cultures and antibiotic administration met specified standards. Other teams evaluated the need for distinct pneumonia paths for various severity groups and standing orders for when subspecialty consults should occur. All of these interventions led to significant improvement in Forbes's overall clinical results and costs. Forbes went from being a low performer to a high performer within the MedisGroups data base for this diagnosis (see Table 3.1).

Some would argue that MedisGroups was designed for indicator tracking for external customers interested in selective contracting, not continuous improvement. The resolution of that debate is beyond the scope of this book. The MedisGroups system has undergone significant changes over the past several years, including new product development. The Forbes project appeared to be motivated by the comparative performance data, but the improvement work required collection and use of additional process data generated outside the MedisGroups data base. Most of the data used in this quality improvement project required primary data collection.

The successes for Forbes Health System are noteworthy. Not only did Forbes improve patient outcomes and cost containment, it enrolled many clinicians in the quality program, adding momentum by its accomplishments. Forbes staff members took some risks

Table 3.1. Pneumonia Project Findings.

| Variable | Before | After |
|---|---|---|
| ER blood cultures | 36% | 96% |
| ER sputum cultures | 53 | 86 |
| Antibiotics < 4 hours | 42 | 87 |
| Mortality rate | 10.2 | 6.8 |
| Average length of stay | 10.4 days | 9.1 days |

Source: © Quality Review Bulletin 19(4). Oakbrook Terrace, IL: Joint Commission on Accreditation of Healthcare Organizations, 1993, p. 127. Reprinted with permission.

to discover how TQM could be used in their setting and found it developed their own abilities to use the skills effectively.

## Management of Stroke Patients: Rehabilitation Institute of Chicago

This story demonstrates the importance of evaluating the cost-benefit of process changes before investing in major organizational restructuring (Falconer and others, 1993). The Rehabilitation Institute evaluated the potential impact of a proposed change in its care process for stroke patients. It wanted to determine whether critical pathways could be used to achieve better outcomes and lower costs. Patients were randomized to the "usual care" of a multidisciplinary care approach and "experimental care" based on an individualized care path, patient treatment goals, and integrated interdisciplinary approach (see Figure 3.4). The two approaches to care involved the same professionals working together in different ways. They compared patients at discharge and at twelve months for their survival, functional status, and other outcomes of interest.

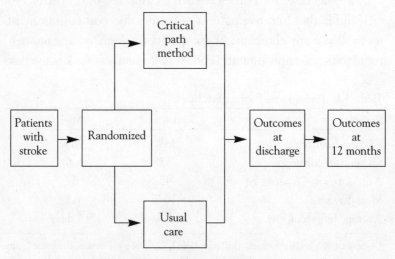

Figure 3.4. Randomized Clinical Trial Study Design.
Source: © Quality Review Bulletin 19(1), Oakbrook Terrace, IL: Joint Commission on Accreditation of Healthcare Organizations, 1993, p. 10. Reprinted with permission.

This project was a success because of its design and the fact that a cross-functional group of practitioners from various disciplines worked together to study two approaches to their work. They evaluated the cost-benefit of a proposed process change. They found no significant differences in outcomes between the usual care group and the experimental group.

One explanation for this, as identified in an editorial about the project (Luttman, 1993), is that pathways can only stabilize a process. They are a tool to reduce variation in practice. In this case, the critical path method did not appear to change how practitioners approached their stroke patients. The tool was not used to change behavior. Care paths are a tool to display, train, and monitor a process, but they do not determine which care process works best. To answer that question, one must identify process deficiencies that warrant improvement, generate and test theories of causes of deficiencies, and finally identify remedies or process changes that will reduce process deficiencies. A number of these steps were underdeveloped in this project. The problem exemplifies a common challenge for medical managers: the tools and techniques of quality improvement and planning must be used to discover *how* to change a process to improve efficiency and patient outcomes.

The success of this project was its scientific approach and the fact that the critical-path method was evaluated before widespread implementation. Many organizations approach paths as a panacea without a plan for evaluating their impact on patient outcomes, cost, and practitioners (American Health Consultants, 1993). Quality management is expensive. It can increase effectiveness if used wisely. Judgment about how and when to deploy administrative resources is a key medical management skill.

## Purchaser-Provider Partnerships: Cleveland Health Quality Choice

This project is a success story on many counts. Over the past several years, employers, physicians, and hospitals worked together in the Cleveland area to measure outcomes of care (Shaller, Pine, Naessens, and Ballard, 1992). The project identified state-of-the-art methods to measure mortality, satisfaction, and cost. The goals of the project were to create market-area sophistication about information on quality and to provide this information to the public, after a period of confidential release to hospitals. All key stakeholder groups are represented on the governing board, including employers, hospitals, and physicians. Cleveland is a market with low penetration by managed care, and one interest group not currently involved is payers and managed-care organizations.

The project team began by evaluating existing risk-adjusted outcomes measurement tools available commercially and in the public domain. Based on this review they selected two tools and contracted for the development of a third to provide them with risk-adjusted satisfaction, LOS, mortality, and cost per case. There was a two-year investment of time and resources to ensure the output of the measurement projects would be as accurate and fair as possible.

Enrolling hospitals was challenging and at times contentious (D. Harper, personal communication, 1994). Although their participation is voluntary, they are under tremendous pressure to measure and report publicly their comparative performance on the Cleveland Choice project measures. Extensive education to providers, purchasers, and the media prepared all interested parties for appropriate interpretation of the data before the project was ready for implementation. There are regular users' meetings to review problems and refine the tools. Data are collected from medical records, abstractors are trained and monitored by the independent organization, and there is a formal audit for data integrity. Hospitals and businesses share in the cost of building and running the system.

Public release of the information did not occur until hospitals had a one-year period to respond to the findings internally. Performance ratings are released twice a year and the project is ongoing. Purchasers who want to use the detailed information about hospitals are required to participate in a full-day training in data analysis and statistics. The media have participated in this train-ing process as well. Hospitals can pull out of the project if they choose. Over thirty hospitals continue to participate on an ongo-ing basis. The successes for this project include the rigorous approach to measurement design and implementation, the open participatory nature of the process, and the emphasis on training users of the results.

Time will tell what impact the project has on the quality of care delivered to Cleveland residents and on the market dynamics in the area. It is yet to be determined how significantly the data from this project will be used to improve care or to inspire in-depth projects that lead to improvement. A summary "report card" (see Table 3.2) is available through local pharmacies because the demand was too great to be handled by direct mail. There is already evidence that the information is being used to make purchasing decisions between health plans and hospitals. The project is recognized as one of the most substantive, albeit aggressive, customer-supplier partnerships in the country.

## Quality in Private Practice: Asthma Home Care Program (AHCP)

This story exemplifies how TQM applies to private office practice and the potential impact on patients (Johnson, 1992). It is one of

Table 3.2. Report Card: Hospital Patient Satisfaction.

| Performance measure | Global satisfaction | Total process |
|---|---|---|
| Satisfaction higher than predicted | Hospitals A, C, D, M | Hospitals C, E, G, S |
| Satisfaction as predicted | 22 hospitals | 17 hospitals |
| Satisfaction lower than predicted | Hospitals B, F, O, T | Hospitals D, H, J, T, U, V, W, Z |

a number of examples of quality projects that clinicians have done independent of any specific training or infrastructure called TQM. It manifests many important TQM principles and techniques and demonstrates just how much TQM and clinical practice have in common.

An allergist with a large population of patients with asthma began experimenting with specified treatment protocols in the early 1980s. He developed acute-care protocols for emergency office visits to standardize the management of asthmatic patients who presented with acute exacerbations. While this appeared anecdotally to improve outcomes of acute episodes, patients had difficulty maintaining the regimen because they found it difficult to remember how to take their medications and lost interest when their symptoms subsided.

To solve this problem, the physician developed a chart for patients to use in monitoring their symptoms and drug use over time; the goal was to help them manage their own illness. From 1984 to 1987, he worked with his patients, eliciting their feedback in refining the design of the chart so it would be easy for them to use. The final chart identifies three color-coded clinical status zones: green, yellow, and red (Figure 3.5). Patients were instructed to take peak flow readings at home when they felt symptomatic, record them on the chart, and take their medications per their home care program. In case of severe acute symptoms, patients were instructed to call for emergency help and follow the red-zone instructions. Over several years, patients were managed with this system. In 1991, a similar type of tricolor chart with patient-care instructions was recommended by the National Asthma Education Program practice guideline (National Heart, Lung and Blood Institute, 1991).

In 1992, the practitioner did a retrospective analysis to evaluate the impact of the home care program. One hundred and thirty-six cases of asthma managed before and after the program were compared to determine the incidence of acute-care episodes and relative costs. Patients were surveyed to assess their satisfaction and

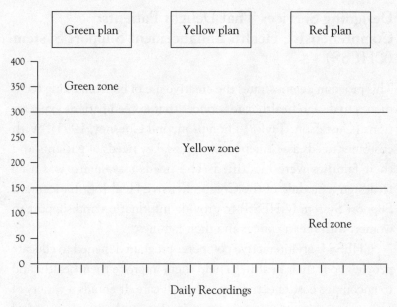

Figure 3.5. Asthma Home Care Program.

compliance with the program. While the design of this analysis cannot prove causality with the certainty of a randomized controlled trial, the findings were suggestive. Analyses showed an 81 percent decrease in hospitalizations, 92.4 percent decrease in emergency room visits, 11.8 percent increase in emergency office visits, and 2.4 percent increase in routine office visits for asthma. The average cost per patient per year dropped 60.6 percent, and 87 percent of patients were satisfied with the program. While functional outcomes were not measured, the reduced rates of acute episodes is an indirect measure of patient function.

This initiative is an example of applied science in routine clinical practice. It demonstrates how individual practitioners can focus on cohorts of patients with comparable diagnoses and severity, design innovative management plans, evaluate them, and improve them over time. This program further demonstrates the type of innovation that is possible when practitioners listen to patients and involve them in their own care.

## Designing Services That Delight Patients: Comprehensive Health Enhancement Support System (CHESS)

This program demonstrates the creative use of benchmarking techniques to design health care services that exceed patient expectations (Gustafson, Taylor, Thompson, and Chesney, 1993). With customer needs assessment techniques, key needs of patients and their families were identified. The needs assessment was used to design a module of the Comprehensive Health Enhancement Support System (CHESS) to provide information and support to women with breast cancer and their families.

CHESS is an interactive computer program designed to educate people about their health, to help them improve their health, and to encourage cost-effective use of health care. It entails a variety of sources of information, including questions and answers, personal stories, data base on articles, electronic mail "Ask an Expert," information about support groups, and many other features.

The effort to build a breast cancer module of CHESS began with designing a survey instrument to elicit needs of patients, their partners, and their daughters. They used Delphi process (Dalkey and Helmer, 1967), nominal group process (Delbecq, 1975), and other tools to capture diverse ideas and organize them systematically. The needs assessment was used to develop a survey instrument for each of the three customer groups. After surveys were tested and administered to samples, data were analyzed to gain a full understanding of the needs. This analysis was used to design new programs in CHESS.

After the breast cancer module was operational, CHESS was evaluated in a pilot study. Nearly 80 percent of women accepted placement of a CHESS computer in their home and used the module several times a day for three months. Women of all ages and education levels found CHESS useful. Clinicians from the University Hospital in Madison were so pleased that they now make CHESS available to all breast cancer surgery patients.

This program is a prototype in a number of ways. It demonstrates the potential applications in health care for surveys and market research techniques. These techniques are underutilized in clinical practice and they open a wealth of opportunities to create patient-focused care. Finally, the breast cancer module of CHESS was designed to allow for evaluation of the program's value for patients and their families. Building self-evaluation into the design of clinical care programs is of critical importance.

## Mammography Screening in an HMO: Harvard Community Health Plan (HCHP)

HCHP's mammography screening project was one of the earliest examples of TQM approaches applied to clinical processes (Platt, 1991). It began in 1989 with data showing that there was substantial variation in the rate of completion of mammography screening in different health centers at HCHP. The quality council chartered a cross-functional team to improve the mammography screening rate for women over forty who visit internal medicine.

The team's first step was to review a random sample of charts to determine what characterizes women who do not get mammograms and why they do not get this early disease detection service (see Figure 3.6). They discovered that most visitors who did not get a mammogram did not have one ordered. They generated a number of hypotheses about why this happened: doctors do not believe mammograms are necessary, patients do not believe mammograms are safe, patients are afraid mammograms are painful, patients do not have their own doctors, and so on.

The team then tested these hypotheses by interviewing patients and physicians. They discovered that women who made acute-care visits but did not have a screening checkup did not get mammograms because they assumed someone would inform them if they needed one. Alternatively, physicians did not feel they had time during acute-care visits to schedule mammograms and were ambivalent

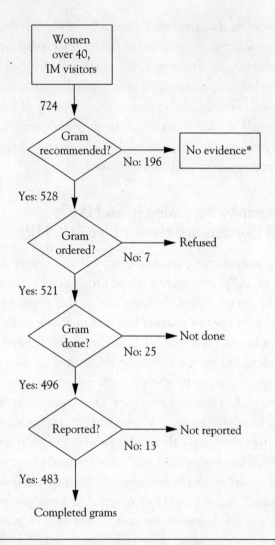

* Most visitors who did not get a mammogram did not have one ordered.

Figure 3.6.  Mammography Screening.

about ordering mammograms on women who had not had annual breast exams. Consequently, women who were not getting screening visits were not having mammograms. These same women who made visits were not receiving any screening or disease prevention care (Pap smears, blood pressure, and other services).

Having determined the root cause of the mammography screening rate, the team moved on to identify which process change would result in the greatest gain in the mammography rate. Several process interventions involving patient education and reminders were proposed and tested. The team compared patient responsiveness to a personal letter from their physician, a letter from the plan medical director stressing the importance of mammography, and a third intervention involving the office staff. The third intervention entailed training and empowering office staff to check patients' medical records for mammography and other screening tests and personal encouragement to schedule a checkup if indicated. The data demonstrated that the third intervention, which relied on personal contact and support, had the greatest impact on screening rates.

On-site mammography was made more easily accessible and the process of notifying patients about the importance of mammography was revised. After two years of work on this issue, the mammography rate increased significantly. Undoubtedly, with a corporate HCHP goal to increase the mammography screening rate, there is a considerable Hawthorne effect involved in the change. There was also tremendous attention to implementing prevention guidelines as a result of a major purchaser initiative that may have had an impact on public and professional awareness and screening rates.

## Purchaser Health Plan Partnership: Massachusetts Healthcare Purchaser Group (MHPG)

These projects have many features in common with the Cleveland Health Quality Choice program described earlier and the national standardized health plan measurement project called the Healthplan

Employer Data and Information Set (HEDIS) (Bloomberg, 1993; National Committee on Quality Assurance, 1994).

The MHPG was organized by purchasers seeking to coordinate a marketwide commitment to cost containment, quality improvement, performance measurement, and public disclosure of information. Representing more than twenty-five large businesses, it was formed in 1993 for the purpose of challenging managed-care organizations to develop a three-year initiative to establish health care quality standards and reduce premiums.

The MHPG Quality Challenge requested that managed-care plans report publicly by January 1994 on six indicators of health care that represent some basic aspect of quality of care provided to health plan members: rate of prenatal care within the first trimester, asthma admission rate, cesarean section rate, hypertension screening rate, mammography screening rate, and mental health days per patient-year. The reports on quality of care were intended to provide a baseline performance profile for each of the health plans.

The MHPG quality measures were designed during 1990, 1991, and 1992 by quality professionals representing three of the twenty plans participating in the Quality Challenge. The selected measures are very similar to some of the HEDIS measures simultaneously under development by a national task force of purchasers and health plans, including representatives from Massachusetts. The HEDIS measures are widely acknowledged as minimalist, to allow all plans a chance to meet the measurement expectations. Both MHPG and HEDIS measurement initiatives were forced by the pragmatic concerns and the cost of measurement to keep their indicators simple.

The purpose of the MHPG Cost Challenge was to constrain premium increases to no more than 4 percent above the consumer price index (CPI). The hope was to control health benefit expense by limiting managed-care organizations' premium increases to no more than 1 percent above the CPI by 1997. This is expected to lead to increased discounts to providers, greater selective contracting with cost-effective providers, and increased sharing of financial risk with providers as well as better resource management by providers.

In the early phase of the MHPG project, the goal was to address feasibility and logistical obstacles to accurate measurement and reporting. As the project came to completion and was reported in a comprehensive document in March 1994, the purchaser community wanted to take the next step and use the data to make comparisons. Like the Cleveland project, significant effort went toward educating purchasers and the press about the problems with measurement in its infancy. Repeated cautions about data quality and completeness has dampened the market's enthusiasm for making buying decisions with the data in the short run. This caution may be justified today but plans recognize that prudent purchasing based on reported performance is around the corner.

The New England HEDIS Coalition built on the MHPG project's success. It is a broader-based group actively involving scores of employer and health plan representatives in a coordinated initiative to use HEDIS measures in the Massachusetts market. Together, large teams undertook to apply the HEDIS measures to fifteen competing health plans. Employers focused on learning the complexity of such measurement, including the need for severity adjustment.

These two thriving organizations and their projects are a success in terms of the level of purchaser and health plan involvement. They mark the first time that collaboration in a large geographic market area has led to widespread generation and use of data. Similar projects are under way in other regions, including Texas and California. These projects exemplify a lesson learned in many regions previously: when purchasers combine forces and speak with a common voice, they can be much more successful in fostering healthy competition and collaboration among plans.

These projects also spawned a broad network of purchasers, health plans, health services researchers, and public agencies engaged in a constructive dialogue about public disclosure of performance information within the Massachusetts market. In 1994,

Massachusetts witnessed healthy debate on the multitude of questions raised by health plan report cards and provider profiling. While many issues need to be raised and debated, the right interests are at the table seeking to find win-win solutions for the health of the citizens of Massachusetts.

Another positive outcome is the initiation of best-practices conferences among participating health plans. In the spring of 1994, representatives of several plans came together to discuss their care processes in prenatal care and obstetrics. This conference was sponsored by the purchasers, demonstrating their commitment to creating a feedback loop (see Figure 3.7) and fostering continuous improvement.

For any purchaser-provider partnerships, it is important to continually self-assess the breadth and depth of the effort. Projects focused only on cost or any other narrow perspective will have a limited impact. It is important to check the "control panel" (see Figure 3.8) to be sure that performance indicators cover all aspects of value in health care.

## Conclusion

Significant progress has been made in recent years in applying sophisticated management techniques to health care settings. In

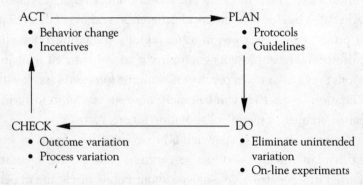

Figure 3.7. Feedback Loop.

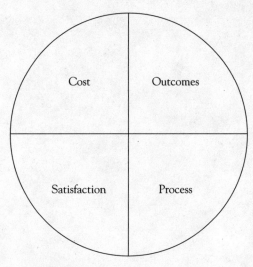

Figure 3.8.  Control Panel.

general, greater progress has been demonstrated in the contained environment of the hospital than in the ambulatory setting, as demonstrated by the examples in this chapter. With the rapid move to vertical integration within the health care industry and increasing pressure on health plans in general, it is likely that this balance will shift over the next five to ten years. Increasingly, there will be examples that span the entire episode of illness, independent of institutional boundaries.

These stories are provided as food for thought. They are concrete examples of TQM tools and techniques applied to clinical care. The next three chapters focus on specific tools and techniques.

# 4

. . . . . . . . . . . . . . . . . . . . . . . . . . . . .

# Measuring Care and
# Managing Variation

There is a popular phrase to describe a simple lesson in quality management: "You can't manage what you can't measure!" This rule applies to clinical practice as well to other professions and industries. The challenge for clinicians and health services researchers is finding valid, reliable, and cost-efficient methods to measure practice and outcomes.

Medical managers need diagnostic tools to assess quality just as practitioners need cultures to identify bacteria. To improve clinical practice, tools are needed that can diagnose root causes of process deficiencies. The sensitivity and specificity of these tools must be known, as with any other diagnostic tool. An even bigger challenge may be to define the appropriate use of quality-of-care measures (Kassirer, 1993).

## Measurement's Role in TQM

Within the Juran Trilogy of quality management approaches (see Table 1.1), measurement plays a role in control, improvement, and planning. In fact, Juran has stated that the P-D-C-A (plan, do, check, act) cycle of improvement should begin with the check (measurement) step. Otherwise, the focus of improvement efforts may be misguided. Unless data drive priorities for quality management, TQM will have limited impact on performance or market share. Data collection should be built into the course of caring for patients. Medical managers need to continually ask, Who needs the information and how will it be used? Toward what goal?

Measurement is a major source of frustration for organizations implementing quality programs in clinical practice. At its core, this frustration stems from confusion about the difference between off-line and on-line research (see Figure 2.7). By and large, clinicians are familiar with off-line research directed at discovering new technologies and treatments. Off-line research was the sole focus of the professional literature until recently. On-line measurement, with its focus on outcomes in day-to-day practice, is a new concept for most practitioners. On-line measurement is used to identify assignable variation, investigate root causes of process capability and random variation, and test ways to revise routine process of care. Because it is grounded in epidemiology and operational sciences, it is less familiar.

Not only are the methods of on-line measurement different from efficacy research and quality assurance case review, implementation also is quite different. This measurement activity is not funded by research grants, nor is it billable to payers and purchasers under most circumstances. It is an overhead expense that hits the bottom line for hospitals, managed-care organizations, and integrated systems.

In the absence of clear focus, most measurement activity naturally expands in scope and complexity. Given their limited experience with on-line measurement, some practitioners replicate the approach and complexity of academic research and find themselves overwhelmed. Medical managers face the challenge of introducing new administrative costs for measurement that must be justifiable in this era of cost reduction.

## Why Create Feedback Loops?

Together with financial and other personal incentives, feedback has been shown to be the most effective method of changing physician behavior (Greco and Eisenberg, 1993; McNeil, Pedersen, and Gatsonis, 1992). Guideline promotion, without physician feedback, has inconsistently been shown to influence practice patterns (Berman, 1992; Lomas, 1989). Feedback of data on practice patterns and outcomes (see Figure 4.1) is an effective and constructive method of allowing physicians to reduce unintended practice variation.

This should come as no surprise. Physicians are scientists and are trained to be attentive to data (James, 1989). Clinicians currently function in the dark—in a black box, so to speak. They have little information available to tell them how well their patients, in aggregate, are doing. When data are provided, clinicians respond.

If you ask a room full of pediatricians, "What percentage of your two-year-old patients have been immunized according to national standards?" you will usually get one of two answers: "I don't know" or "All of them!" If you ask how they know all of them have been immunized, the response is often, "Because I immunized them!" Behind this answer is a heartfelt statement of intention. All pediatricians want to immunize the children in their practice according

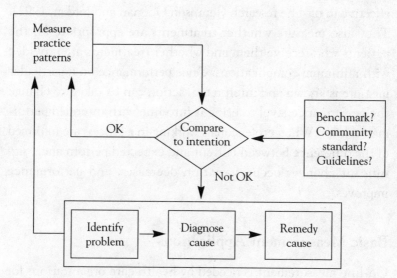

Figure 4.1. Feedback Loops.

to national standards of good practice. But the more important question is, "How many children actually get immunized and how many are on schedule?" The answer may have little to do with anyone's intention and everything to do with processes and how well they are designed and functioning.

You can ask a similar question to any group of specialists. To a group of internists: "What percentage of your hypertensive patients are controlled? What percentage of your diabetics have had an ophthalmology visit?" To a group of gynecologists: "What percentage of your hysterectomies were indicated as defined by national guidelines?" Today, virtually no group of specialists can tell you about the rate at which they achieve optimal outcomes for their patients. "How long, on average, does it take your patients to return to work after a myocardial infarction? After a total hip replacement?" This type of information should be an entitlement for physicians but, at present, feedback information is not available, and data that are available tend to be irrelevant to clinicians.

On-line measurement and feedback are designed to measure whether practitioners use treatment modalities that have proven effective in off-line research (Jennison Goonan and Jordan, 1992). They also measure whether treatments are appropriate for the patients who receive them and whether treatments are provided with minimum complications. Once performance on a particular measure is known and interpreted, action can be taken to change the performance level to bring it into line with intended performance level. When professionals working in a process are informed of the difference between current and expected performance, significant changes occur, variation decreases, and performance improves.

## Basic Measurement Applications

On-line measurement is needed by health care organizations for three general management activities:

1. Process improvement

2. Aggregate practice pattern analysis

3. High-level performance tracking

Each serves different yet related purposes. It helps to understand the role of each type of measurement and the techniques needed to fulfill each purpose.

*Measurement for improvement* is the relatively targeted measurement conducted to diagnose process deficiencies and pilot-test proposed process changes to enhance performance. These are data collected by cross-functional teams chartered to solve a specific problem within a set time frame. Typically, these on-line experiments require simple data collection and analysis (Gaucher and Coffey, 1993). They are not designed to compare outside the organization or for external reporting. Data for improvement must be easy to collect, interpret, and act upon. Its purpose is to inform members of an improvement team how and where to change the process of care. Typically, data are collected to test theories of cause or pilot process changes (see Chapter Seven). Such data are unlikely to produce new knowledge about effectiveness of medical practice or to prove the efficacy of a treatment. These data may be of interest to other organizations but may not be sufficiently rigorous to produce generalizations about optimal practice.

*Data for Improvement*

- Simple short-term data collection

- Focused topic or question

- Relation to specific process improvement

- Minimal statistical sophistication

The second type of measurement activity relates to using or creating data bases to analyze *aggregate practice patterns* and feed information back to practitioners. The users of these data are clinical leaders and practitioners who seek comparative information about their practice patterns. Health plans also use this type of data to compare practitioners' practice patterns. Many purchasers demand that health plans distribute analyses of administrative data bases as feedback, called practice profiles. A number of commercial vendors license systems for this purpose (The MedStat Group, GMIS, Value Health Sciences, and others).

Some health care organizations have invested in developing comprehensive data bases for general use in quality improvement initiatives (Curtis, 1994), reimbursement programs (Minnesota Blue Cross/Blue Shield), and public reporting (Pennsylvania Cost Containment Council, 1992). For these projects, data are generated by primary data collection from the medical record. These projects produce clinical data bases that are analyzed to report comparative performance as well as produce feedback to providers.

*Aggregate Practice Analysis*

- Administrative data to reveal practitioner patterns

- Primary data to address quality-of-care issues

- Intended use for comparative analysis

- Partially risk-adjusted data

The third type of measurement activity focuses on *summary performance reporting*. This sort of measurement serves the needs of top management that needs a "control panel" on the performance of the organization as a whole. These data are used to inform organizational strategic planning. Purchasers increasingly demand evidence of performance tracking. The types of measures in this category are summary indicators on performance in quality of care, cost, productivity, and innovation. Few health care organizations have such a tracking system in place or are in a position to monitor themselves against such measures. Cutting-edge institutions are moving in this direction. Indicators and reporting for this purpose must be coordinated with measurement for improvement. Indicators should address topics that providers can affect. Improvement against the measures should correlate with better outcomes.

The more common initiative in this arena is known as a report card—summary performance tracking imposed by purchasers on health plans and providers (Mitka, 1993). There are numerous examples of hospitals and health plans using report cards to demonstrate their value to prospective purchasers (Bloomberg, 1993; Shaller, Pine, Naessens, and Ballard, 1992). This area of measurement activity is in rapid evolution, particularly in view of its potential use and abuse. External customers have a right to expect comparable performance information on institutional and plan-level performance. Issues surrounding standardization of measurement and audit of the data will get resolved over the next several years. Regardless of these efforts to provide information on performance to external customers, top leadership of health systems need to have comprehensive, summarized performance information to help them steer the organization's internal improvement program.

### Summary Performance Tracking

- High-level indicators of competitive performance

- Indicators for important aspects of care and key diagnoses

- Top-leadership monitoring and planning

- Report cards for purchasers

In the future, all three types of measurement activities will fit together in a multipurpose program of health care information for health plans and systems. Certainly some aggregate practice pattern analyses and summary performance indicators foster quality improvement. There is some gain in performance simply by "turning the lights on" and feeding information on performance to practitioners. But the major gains, the breakthroughs in performance, come from identifying root causes and key drivers in a scientific manner or redesigning care processes through creative planning. Likewise, some information generated by improvement teams can inform senior leadership about the organization's overall performance. Generally speaking, however, each of the three measurement types will require several more years before they fit nicely together into a comprehensive measurement system (Nadzam, 1991).

The Joint Commission on Accreditation of Healthcare Organizations (JCAHO) promotes a model for assessing care that highlights the complexity of this challenge (see Figure 4.2). The "quality cube" shows that there are three dimensions to address in a comprehensive measurement system: the basic management functions that should be present in any quality organization, dimensions of performance relevant to health care, and patient populations specific to a particular organization (Schyve, 1994). Ultimately, measurement must be developed for all three applications.

For today's medical manager, measurement and its implementation to meet all customers and their needs can be overwhelming. Knowing the customers of the information and understanding their intended use of it can inform careful planning in this critical area.

## Measurement for Improvement

Measurement for improvement focuses on common, easily defined cohorts of patients and relatively straightforward aspects of their care. Performing this type of data collection requires more common sense than research experience. The data collection should be simple to administer, preferably by clinicians as they make their usual records and notes. The analysis should use simple tools such as histograms and scatter diagrams. The project results are measured in change in practice patterns and desired outcomes, not in the number of publications in the literature.

Recall the story of Medical Center Hospital of Vermont described in Chapter Three. The team used process steps in the

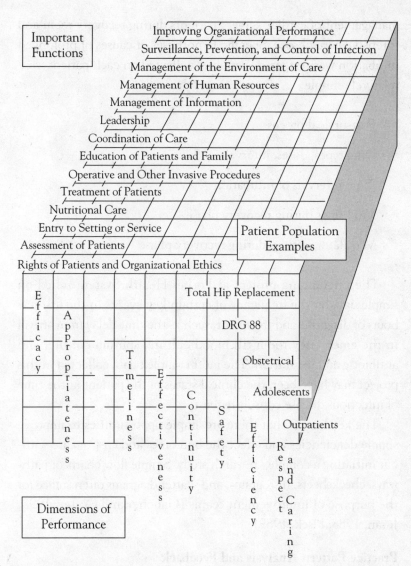

Figure 4.2. The Quality Cube: A Model for Assessing the Quality of Health Care.

*Source:* © 1995 *Comprehensive Accreditation Manual for Hospitals.* Oakbrook Terrace, Ill.: Joint Commission on Accreditation of Healthcare Organizations. Reprinted with permission.

management of cardiac surgery patients during recovery room and intensive care phases. Specific hypotheses of causes of prolonged intubation were targeted. Variables collected on each patient were relatively simple:

Postsurgical process

Drug types, doses, intervals

Time intervals of intubation

Vital signs during recovery phase

Ventilator settings during recovery phase

The pneumonia project at Forbes Health System relied on simple data on the frequency of certain key events in the first few hours of diagnosis and treatment, such as the time delay from arrival in the emergency room till blood culture, sputum culture, and antibiotic administration. The most complex data collected in this project may have been the clinical status of the patient at the time of infectious disease consult request.

The key here is that there are ample opportunities to improve simple deficiencies and affect the outcomes and cost of care without initiating a complex research study. Simple flow charts or pathways, checksheets, histograms, and scatter diagrams often suffice for the purpose of improvement teams (Gaucher and Coffey, 1993; Juran, 1988; Plsek, 1989).

## Practice Pattern Analysis and Feedback

Juran defined quality control as measuring key processes, assessing variation in performance, and reducing variation that is unintended or counterproductive. Quality control activities in the health care arena include data analysis and feedback to the people who work in care processes. A feedback loop provides information to practitioners about their practice patterns. It is generally informative to make a number of comparisons such as one organization's or one individual's practice over time. Other comparisons can also be useful, such as physician to peer group, institution to institution, and so on. Comparisons help inform the next step—judging whether the results of measurement indicate a need to change practice patterns.

Aggregate practice analysis and feedback can also focus healthy discussion among practitioners about best demonstrated practices, leading to reduction in variation. As has been shown by organizations that implement measurement and feedback, practice patterns change substantially when information is provided to clinicians (James, Horn, and Stephenson, 1994). As part of a study done at Intermountain Health Care, data on prophylactic antibiotic administration and deep postoperative wound infection rates were fed back to surgeons. The data base was collected as part of a nonrandomized prospective study of practice patterns of antibiotic use and outcomes. Feedback resulted in a drop in the postsurgical wound infection rate from 1.8 percent to 0.9 percent, a rate that continued to decline (Classen, Evans, and Pestonik, 1992).

Feedback of aggregate practice data to hospitals or practitioners can reduce variation in their practice patterns (see Figure 4.3). Reduction in variation brings a process into control or stabilizes it. Practitioners are unaware of their own practice variation and naturally reduce it substantially when provided information. This type of feedback and control or stabilization is a prerequisite for significant innovation and improvement. It is virtually impossible to identify root cause of poor performance of a care process riddled with unintended variation. Breakthroughs in performance occur when process is in control and on-line experiments can be conducted to identify innovative process designs.

Another example of successful feedback loops was developed by the Connecticut Hospital Association, which implemented a voluntary program linking various data bases and generated a set of indicators including hospital-specific mortality rates for acute myocardial infarction. The feedback loop identified hospitals with

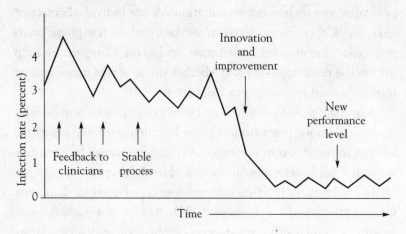

Figure 4.3. How Feedback Affects Performance.

opportunities to improve. The indicators triggered improvement projects and targeted data collection to identify how and where to change the care process.

The key to successful feedback loops is to minimize judgment of performance and maximize the informative nature of the feedback. To accomplish this, practitioners must be viewed as the customer of the feedback process and the analyses must be designed according to their needs and requirements.

There is a burgeoning industry of software vendors who take administrative data from hospitals and health plans and generate practice profiles for feedback, strategic planning, quality planning, and other uses. Profiling should meet basic research standards for accuracy if it is to be used in any meaningful way (Kassirer, 1994).

## Measurement for Summary Performance Reporting

The major customers of this type of measurement activity are the senior leaders of hospitals and managed-care organizations, regulators, and purchasers and their consultants. Report card initiatives in Pennsylvania and Cleveland are examples. The emerging Indicator Measurement System of the JCAHO is intended to specify measures useful for this purpose. Monitoring the performance of health systems on a set of key, summary indicators will become a routine task for quality improvement professionals in the future. At Blue Cross and Blue Shield of Massachusetts, the director of medical policy, evaluation, and improvement presents semiannual updates to a subcommittee of the board of directors. Most health plans in the country will soon be reviewing their performance against the HEDIS 2.0 data set (standardized measures of health plan performance) or challenged to complete it (Corrigan and Nielson, 1993). St. Louis and Massachusetts have undergone an evaluation published in publications called *Health Pages*. These magazines highlight physicians, hospitals, and health plans in a consumer guide format (Schneider, 1993).

Summary performance information is relevant to clinical leaders and practitioners but usually only because it focuses attention and directs improvement efforts (Nerenz, 1993). Indicators rarely highlight *how* to change the process of care. For example, every health plan in the country should have improvement efforts under way to improve some aspect of care to patients with coronary artery disease. This topic rises to the top of every list of areas for improvement because it is so common and costly in any adult population. But what aspect of care should be improved? HEDIS 2.0 includes population-based cardiac catheterization and surgery rates. While the correct rates are unknown, health plans that vary widely from local and national norms are wise to demonstrate results improving the rate of *appropriateness* of these procedures in their population. To have impact on the rate of appropriateness, different measurement and improvement tools at a greater level of detail are required.

In the Massachusetts market, the purchaser community has demonstrated a long-term view of how performance profiles should be used. The primary objective is to drive improvement by (1) asking questions, (2) requiring action, and (3) assessing impact. The *Boston Globe* reported that these data are preliminary and should not be used for purchasing decisions for a year or two (Stein, 1994).

Ultimately, both purchasers and health care organization senior leadership need a set of indicators to monitor, rather like a control panel. Through tracking performance over time (see Figure 4.3), health care organizations go beyond identifying what needs improvement to monitoring the impact of improvement initiatives. Measurement at one point in time can be a random incident. Annualized rates can be equally misleading because they lack the detail of a time trend. By tracking indicators over time, we can distinguish between assignable causes and chronic, random variation and make sound management decisions about the best response to performance information.

Let common sense guide priorities. Purchasers expect the obvious:

- They expect rates of preventable complications to be measured and eliminated. Though they are extremely interested in long-term functional outcomes, they realize that these applications are somewhat experimental today. Meanwhile, neglecting preventable nosocomial infections or surgical complications is analogous to airlines neglecting ice on the wings at take-off: there are obvious hazards that should be prevented.

- Measures of efficiency and financial stability are crucial in today's market. Both health plans and purchasers are interested in partnerships with cost-efficient, secure organizations, selling at the lowest price that does not threaten quality of care.

- Patient access and satisfaction are clearly important for measurement. Today, they determine consumer choice.

- It is important to demonstrate an organization's ability to innovate in patient-focused care. Successful organizations will demonstrate breakthrough performance in their ability to design patient-centered services tailored to targeted patient populations.

Customers, particularly large employer-purchasers and accreditation organizations, expect hospitals and HMOs to make every effort to adjust outcome measures for risk. They expect measurement to be ongoing and to monitor the impact of quality improvement activities. Without feedback loops in place, tracking performance over time will not demonstrate improvement.

## Obstacles to Measurement

The obstacles to quality measurement boil down to three major issues: accuracy, risk adjustment, and cost. The first two are intricately related. The degree to which quality of care is controllable by providers and the corollary issue, intrinsic patient risk for bad outcomes, are issues that have challenged health services researchers for decades (Iezzoni, 1994c).

### Accuracy

The purposes of designing and applying indicators of quality are to evaluate the performance of clinical care and to generate actionable information for improvement. Crucial to these purposes is the accuracy of the measures. There are several ways to assess the accuracy of a measurement method or test: validity, reliability, sensitivity, specificity, clinical relevance, and so forth. These apply to indicators of quality as well as to any other measurement, yet rarely are these characteristics defined for quality indicators.

Even more fundamental is the fact that many factors affect the accuracy of measures of quality and effectiveness. The degree to which outcomes result from clinical decisions and the process of care is unknown. Patient attributes, patient preferences, and flaws in the data retrieved from claims, medical records, and surveys all contribute to imprecision in measurement (Guadagnoli and McNeil, 1994).

These issues of accuracy are critically important for public policy and purchasing decisions based on measurement. They are less important for internal improvement activities, where accuracy of comparisons does not require the same level of certainty. Both external and internal applications of performance information benefit greatly from enhanced accuracy. This remains a hope for the future for most organizations.

## Risk Adjustment

Risk adjustment builds on the epidemiologic concept of risk. Patients with certain similar characteristics are at comparable risk of an adverse outcome such as tumor recurrence or mortality. Tracking outcomes and relating them to the processes of care can be accomplished only if factors beyond the control of physicians are identified and taken into account in the design of measurements (Iezzoni, 1989, 1991). The epidemiologic concept of risk includes the idea of "severity of illness," meaning the level of severity of a particular condition. One patient may have mild pneumonia while another has severe pneumonia. It also includes the concept of "case mix," which typically refers to the presence or absence of comorbid conditions, which affect an individual patient's overall risk of adverse outcomes.

Finally, there is risk, perhaps the most generic concept. It refers to the notion that there are underlying patient characteristics, including severity and comorbidities, that influence the risk or probability of various outcomes of interest. Regardless of what term we use, the goal is to identify a measurement method that allows for meaningful, accurate, and informative comparison of groups of patients. No risk adjustment method is perfect.

### Stratification Versus Risk Adjustment

There are two basic strategies used to make patients comparable to one another, allowing us to compare outcomes in populations of patients. These two strategies are stratification and risk adjustment, and they can be used separately or in conjunction with one another.

Stratification is something clinicians do naturally when thinking about patients. It simply refers to grouping patients with other patients with similar diagnoses and intrinsic risk for various outcomes, such as complications, mortality, functional status, or total cost. Diagnostic related groups (DRGs) are a stratification method designed to group patients into categories so that they are comparable in terms of their probability of overall inpatient resource use. In this case, resource use is the outcome for which the method is designed to optimize predictability.

Consider some clinical examples. When thinking about clinical outcomes for patients with asthma, it is helpful to stratify patients into smokers and nonsmokers because this characteristic increases the probability of various asthma-related outcomes such as poor respiratory function and total cost of care. In children, it might be useful to stratify on gender, because the disease affects boys and girls differently. Among patients with diabetes, stratification into groups increases the similarity of patients' risk of complications, insulin dependence, and the duration of the diabetes. Among patients with hypertension, stratification according to essential versus nonessential, age, and race helps when judging outcomes of treatment. Age and premorbid physical function level are useful stratifiers when comparing outcomes of patients following total hip replacement. The characteristics we choose to classify patients depend on the outcome being measured.

Risk adjustment is less intuitive to clinicians. It entails using statistical modeling to adjust for differences among patients within a strata, to increase the accuracy when their outcomes are compared. It takes into account known factors that cannot easily be built into stratification, such as the presence of other diagnoses or comorbidities.

It is important to recognize that stratification and risk adjustment cannot completely eliminate the impact of disease severity, comorbidity, or other unidentified factors that affect outcome.

Sometimes they do a rather poor job of correcting for these factors. Expert advice on these issues is usually necessary to ensure that quality measurements are understood for what they do and do not accurately measure.

### When Is Risk Adjustment Important?

It is always important to understand the power of measurements and to have an awareness of the degree of accuracy required, depending upon the purpose of the measure. With measures intended for external reporting and public comparisons, the issue of risk adjustment should be considered carefully (Iezzoni, 1994a, 1994c). Risk adjustment may be necessary for summary performance tracking for clinical topics where senior leadership wants to compare performance to other organizations. Risk adjustment is usually desirable for aggregate practice pattern analysis and interpretation.

Risk adjustment is generally *not* necessary for internal quality improvement. Project-by-project improvement should be directed at a defined stratum of patients who are similar, who experience a comparable process of care, and who have comparable probability of outcomes. As a general rule, if statistical adjustment or other sophisticated statistical techniques are needed, the project is sliding into off-line research or the patient cohort was defined too broadly and includes complex patients whose care needs differ from the average patient.

### Cost of Measurement

The third major obstacle to implementing measurement relates to cost and resource requirements. In states and markets where measurement systems have been mandated, the cost of operating outcomes measurement systems is substantial. On the other hand, survivors of the next several rounds of competition will be organizations who invest in building measurement systems that meet internal and external needs for information. The key is to define a strategy and priorities that will position the organization appropriately for success. Many hospitals and insurance companies have wasted millions in this area as a result of poor strategic decisions.

There are two areas to consider. First is information technology infrastructure. In health care organizations, information systems are typically designed to process transactions and expenditures for billing and payment in a fee-for-service environment. Sometimes they log lab test results. Reengineering information systems to meet real-time needs for interactivity and access to encounter, laboratory, and other data poses a major challenge for hospitals and managed-care organizations. Measurement, analysis of practice patterns, and time trend of data add yet another level of complexity. The need to overhaul information technology and bring it to parity with other industries is tremendous. Yet this need has surfaced at a time when margins are rapidly shrinking and resources for capital investment are severely limited.

The second area to consider is personnel to support a strategic measurement function. Most leading organizations have in-house applied research capabilities or they are part of a larger system that has resources on staff. Most professionals who can lead such functions have academic health services research backgrounds with training in public health, health administration, or statistics. Because of the applied nature of on-line measurement in health care, many researchers with academic backgrounds find the new environment frustratingly imprecise. There are few academic training programs that prepare individuals for the practical challenges of on-line measurement work. On-the-job training for individuals with basic data analysis skills can be as effective as recruiting master's level personnel. Quality assurance professionals can be candidates for medical record abstraction for population-based measurements as well as other analysis tasks. Finally, another skill set useful in an on-line measurement function is writing and marketing. Individuals who can write to a lay audience as well as professional audiences can be very productive in this arena.

### Design Feedback Loops

Creating feedback loops for any and all performance data collected by the organization is an important component of on-line measurement. Feedback loops help practitioners improve quality and efficiency, but they must include enough process detail to be informative, clinically relevant, and actionable. For example, in Pennsylvania, hospitals report only outcomes, such as hospital severity-adjusted mortality rates. These reports identify significant variance from expected mortality rates but provide little or no information about defects in the processes that produced the outcome.

When building feedback loops for internal use with practitioners, hospitals and health plans need to focus on the practitioners' needs for actionable information. The pendulum has swung away from gross summary measures of outcome toward measurement that is condition- or diagnosis-specific and stratified and adjusted for condition-specific patient characteristics. These measures are more accurate and more informative to the clinicians whose performance is being measured. The full complement of measures is needed: outcome, process, and efficiency measures. Unfortunately, there is no list of the definitive measures available today. In fact, the number of indicators and measurement systems continues to mushroom. This state of affairs cannot continue. The question as to which measures are best will be answered in the near future.

### Designing a Feedback Loop

Designing a feedback loop is a five-step process:

1. Identify top diagnoses and core functions that are critical for organization's success.

2. Identify priorities related to strategic goals.

3. Design relevant measure and analyses.

4. Collect and analyze data.

5. Design and distribute brief, graphical, actionable information.

Steps 1 and 2 are completed by the highest cross-specialty leadership group or clinical quality council. This group then charters measurement teams who complete Steps 3, 4, and 5.

## Identifying Top Diagnoses and Functions

The first step in designing a feedback loop entails examining your clinical practice and identifying which diagnosis-specific and diagnosis-independent processes are most important to your hospital, group practice, or HMO customers. Which high-volume, high-cost, high-risk diagnoses and processes are most important to monitor and improve? How does an organization select these processes? By identifying the strategic diagnoses and organizational functions that are critical to the survival of the organization.

*Identifying Top Diagnoses and Functions*

Demands from purchasers

High-volume diagnosis and procedures groups

Average cost per case or episode

Regulatory requirements

Core functions that drive success or failure

## Setting Priorities

Once the top diagnoses, conditions, and care processes have been identified, priorities for measurement can be established. This is a crucial step because organizations naturally focus their improvement initiatives on the topics that have been measured. In short, measurement drives the improvement agenda. Priorities for measurement should link back to strategic, annual, and tactical improvement goals. For example, assume that back pain is the most common condition treated within the third-highest category of expenditure for an HMO, musculoskeletal disorders. This would be considered a top diagnosis and care process. However, is it an appropriate priority this year? Perhaps customers are more concerned about smoking cessation or emergency room use at this time. Topics for measurement should be the topics positioned for improvement initiatives as well as top conditions among the population served by the organization. Table 4.1 shows an example of a simple scoring matrix used to help a quality council set priorities. Each council member would be asked to review the topic proposed for measurement and improvement and score it against selection criteria. More important projects receive higher scores. Using a 1, 3, 9 scoring method generates a greater spread in the results. When council members compile their scores, the final discussion and selection of topics will be more informed by using the matrix analysis.

## Chartering Measurement Teams

To ensure that informative measures are used and reported, teams representing all relevant specialties, professions, and quality management staff knowledgeable about measurement should work together to design and implement measures (Joint Commission, 1991). For example, if an HMO plans to measure effectiveness, efficiency, and patient satisfaction with menopause, the measurement team needs representation from internal medicine, gynecology, and

Table 4.1. Matrix for Setting Priorities.

| Processes | Customer requirements | Clinicians' priorities | Benchmark topics | Potential impact | Total score |
|---|---|---|---|---|---|
| Asthma | 9 | 9 | 9 | 3 | 30 |
| High-risk pregnancy | 9 | 3 | 9 | 9 | 30 |
| Mental health | 9 | 3 | 3 | 1 | 16 |
| Adolescent health | 3 | 1 | 1 | 1 | 6 |
| Prevention | 3 | 9 | 9 | 9 | 30 |

endocrinology. Patients and nurse practitioners should be represented as well.

Typically, measurement teams use clinicians as advisers and consultants and require less of their time than improvement teams. In fact, practitioners are really customers of measurement teams because they need performance information to manage their patient populations. The charge to measurement teams is to meet practitioners' information needs.

## Designing and Implementing Measures

Selecting and designing indicators or measurement points are not dissimilar to designing a research protocol. The distinction is subtle but important. Operational quality measurement is not typically designed with sufficient rigor to prove causal relationships between process of care or interventions and patient outcomes. In operational measurement, the goal is to evaluate whether the care is appropriate and efficient, compared with practices that have been proved effective. The frequency of outcomes such as complication rates or admission rates for chronic diseases can be compared to those of other organizations and their level of performance. The purpose is to evaluate performance, not to prove efficacy or effectiveness of interventions.

The charter to a measurement team should specify precisely the process to be measured. This means specifying the patient characteristics for whom the care process is comparable (stratification criteria) and the process end points (beginning and ending points).

After topics are selected and a measurement team is chartered, the team identifies key process and outcome variables that are valuable to measure (see Figure 4.4). All of these decisions should reflect the high-cost, high-morbidity, high-risk topics, process steps, and outcomes.

## Hospital Example

Consider one example cited in the Joint Commission on Accreditation of Healthcare Organizations' (JCAHO) recent publication,

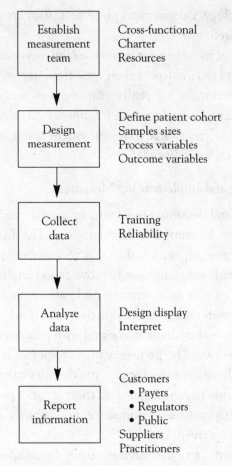

Figure 4.4. Designing and Implementing Measures.

*The Measurement Mandate* (1993b). Obstetrics is one of a hospital's most common and most visible services. An obstetrical department measurement team might choose to measure the effectiveness of the organization in preventing and detecting endometritis in patients following cesarean section. The unit of measure is the patient who develops endometritis within the cohort of patients at risk for the complications: women undergoing cesarean sections (Angelo and Sokol, 1980; Cox and Gilstrap, 1989; Donowitz and Wenzel, 1980). The indicator is expressed as a proportion: the number of women who develop the complication divided by the number of women undergoing the procedure, within a specified time period:

$$\text{Postpartum endometritis rate} = \frac{\text{total number of women with endometritis}}{\text{total number of women undergoing cesarean section}}$$

JCAHO has been developing indicators of hospital quality that will be required as part of the accreditation process beginning in 1996. It is prudent to consider building these indicators into a hospital's quality measurement plan. There are also commercial measurement systems (Maryland Quality Indicators, MedisGroups, APACHE, and others). It is beyond the scope of this book to assess these products. Even when a commercial vendor is selected to assist in quality measurement, significant planning and design work needs to be done by the hospital, group practice, or HMO quality program. Measurement is quite expensive, and it is critical to identify how and why it will be done. Clinicians being measured by such systems need extensive input into the decisions from design to reporting.

## Measurement Design Reports

One tool to consider using is a report that delineates what measures are planned, what they are designed to measure, the rationale and supporting scientific evidence, the sampling techniques, time periods, and uses of the data. This can be used with external customers (purchasers, regulators) as well as internal customers (professionals and staff). Ideally, these reports are limited to one page per topic, as clinicians and purchasers do not have time to study the details. This reporting keeps the relevant people involved so that they are prepared to use information responsibly when it is available. It also helps communicate between customers and suppliers of on-line measurement.

## Interpretation

All measurement is comparative. Few measures have meaning unless they are compared to some other measurement, such as national standards, academy guidelines, internal paths or protocols, benchmark organizations, or competitors.

The actual performance can be measured and interpreted in one of four ways.

1. *Document a level of performance when there is consensus and evidence to support a standard.* An example of this is measurement of the mammography screening rate within the population at risk for breast cancer, specifically women over age fifty. Many HMOs now measure this rate and compare their performance to the established recommendation from the American Cancer Society.

2. *Compare a quality measurement with a peer group caring for comparable patients.* An example of this would be when hospitals compare their complication rates for particular surgeries with other hospitals (see Figure 4.5). When the measurement is comparable

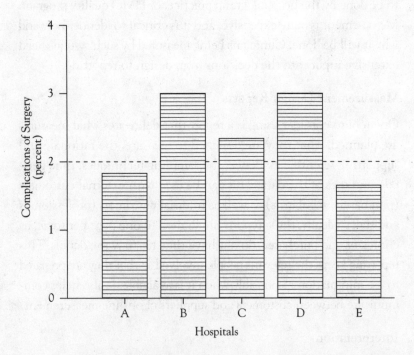

Figure 4.5. Comparison of Risk-Adjusted Outcomes Among Five Peer Hospitals.

and the cases have been risk adjusted, this type of comparison is informative about performance level and potential opportunities to improve.

3. *Use statistical methods to calculate an expected performance level and compare to the observed level using a normative data base.* An example of this would be in communities where hospitals are measuring their mortality rates, adjusting the rates for differences in risk of death among the patients in each hospital, and then comparing the rates to a calculated expected mortality rate (see Figure 4.6).

4. *Analyze the organization's performance over time and display it in a time sequence format.* This method is the most useful and informative, both internally and externally. The control chart approach to the analysis of data (see Figure 4.7) is more powerful than other comparative approaches because it is more informative and yields greater insight (Wheeler, 1993). It provides a basis for interpreting

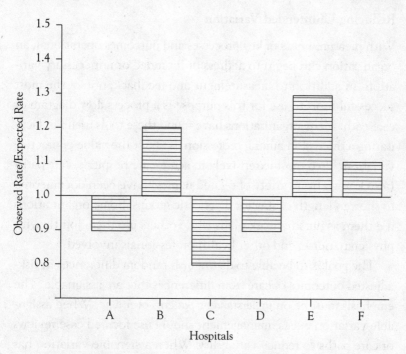

Figure 4.6. Comparison of Mortality Rates, Using Statistical Methods.

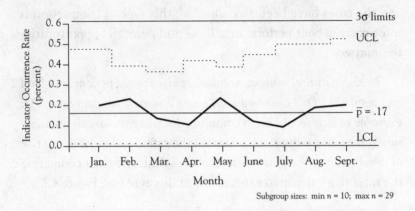

Figure 4.7. Sample Control Chart: Cardiovascular Indicator.

the success of quality improvement efforts and of predicting future performance. It assumes variation will be present. But it allows for distinguishing noise and signals within a data set to guide actions.

## Reducing Unintended Variation

With measurements of key processes and outcomes operational, an organization can begin to address unintended or unnecessary variation. In addition to measurement and feedback, one of the most successful tools to use for this purpose is a process flow diagram or care path. Many organizations have found these tools useful in facilitating a discussion among professionals about the value of practice variation. Used most extensively in acute-care hospitals, care paths (also known by a variety of related names) have been documented to shorten length of stay for diagnostic groups. Some organizations use them as nursing work plans while others use them jointly with physician, nurse, and other health professionals involved.

The goal is to be able to distinguish random differences in risk-adjusted outcomes of care from differences that are assignable. The emphasis must be on *understanding patterns over time*. When assignable variation exists, management should use focused case reviews or care paths to reduce variability. When assignable variation has been largely eliminated and a care process is stable, clinician leaders can decide whether they are satisfied with overall process performance. If they identify important concerns, quality improvement or planning techniques should be employed to redesign the process and achieve better clinical outcomes and efficiency of care.

## Reporting

Regardless of the comparison method your physicians select, you will then need to consider how, when, and to whom to report your results. There are several internal customers who may benefit from routine reporting, and you will also want to consider what type of reports are going to be most useful to them:

Clinicians

Board of directors

Chairs of specialty departments

Quality assurance or management committees

Nursing committee

Ancillary service directors

Payers, employers, and regulators

The decision of whom to share data with must be made with care. Internal customers will need to know that confidentiality of individuals has been protected properly. Keep in mind that physicians do not know that they are practicing differently from their colleagues. They need and deserve assurances that they will not have performance data about their own practices shown to anyone without their permission, except in the situation when a legally mandated reportable event has occurred. Stipulating a set of confidentiality rules and expectations up front will go a long way to build trust within your organization.

The format of reports is important. Quality management reports need to be written so that they are usable by internal and external customers. It will be important to identify the report format needs of the customers of your measurement process. Reports need to be easy to read and understand, without a lot of detail of marginal interest. People have very busy work schedules and often want simple, graphical displays of findings from quality measurements. Typically they want tables of numbers interpreted into concise visual displays that communicate the results. Unlike a journal article or term paper, these reports communicate the bottom line to clinician managers. Backup information about statistical methods and unrevealing preliminary data can be made available on request.

## Evaluating the Measurement Program

When selecting measurements for key diagnoses groups and core organizational functions, it is helpful to use specific criteria to evaluate the utility of measurements. Some criteria for evaluating measures are listed here. These items will help measurement teams stay focused on generating actionable information.

### Evaluating the Measurement Program

1. Clinical relevance of the measure

2. Quality of sources of data

3. Frequency of occurrence

4. Reliability of proposed measure

5. Validity of proposed measure

6. Case mix adjustment or stratification

7. Patient preferences

8. Payer preferences

9. Correlation with other measures or requirements

10. Ability to act on measures for improvement

It is useful to ask measurement teams to evaluate their measurements before and after implementation. This ensures that extraneous data requests are minimized. Similarly, an annual function of the quality council should be to evaluate the effectiveness of the measurement program in general.

## Conclusion

Measurement is a fundamental activity of quality management. It is an area of tremendous frustration and cost for most organizations. Some would argue that it is the major obstacle to managing health care cost and quality. It is also an area of major development and growth. Many issues will be resolved over the next several years, and the obstacles to measurement should diminish as a result.

For now, a thoughtful approach to the selection and use of measurement is in order. Continually provide answers to the questions "How will this information be used, and by whom?" Responsible implementation of measurement and feedback techniques is the key to building a successful quality management program.

# 5

Planning and Designing
Care Processes

Patient outcomes result from an amalgam of patient factors, environmental factors, and factors under the control of practitioners and health care organizations. This last category of controllable factors combines professional decision making with the delivery system's capacity to implement optimal clinical decisions. Often, however, the scientific evidence regarding how best to achieve optimal outcomes for patients is inadequate. All too often clinical practice is based on the old saying "See one, do one, teach one"—as though practicing medicine is a trade rather than an art or a science. The scientific evidence underpinning clinical practice is frequently inadequate or controversial (Eddy, 1990b, 1992).

Furthermore, the clinician's responsibility is to tailor every treatment plan to the unique needs and wants of each individual patient. Patients have different lifestyles and priorities. These differences must be taken into account if we are to achieve optimal outcomes from the patient's perspective. The practitioner's professional obligation is, first and foremost, to meet the individual patient's needs.

These challenges—scientific uncertainty and unique patient needs—enhance the complexity facing clinicians today. They are confounded by expectations from purchasers, managed-care leaders, and public policy makers for minimal variation and documentable uniformity in quality and outcomes of care.

The design tools and techniques of quality planning and customer focus offer practical solutions to these challenges. It is realistic to strive to overcome these obstacles and create a work environment for practitioners that is professionally satisfying as well.

There are two basic applications of design tools and techniques in use for clinical practice today. The first is clinical practice guidelines of all types. Designing and implementing practice guidelines (pathways, algorithms, standing orders, and protocols) provide an avenue to overcome the challenges outlined above. The second application is patient-focused care. Many organizations have redesigned their overall care delivery approach to create a more patient-oriented experience as well as greater efficiency.

## Achieving Results Through Use of Practice Guidelines

While there are many unresolved issues surrounding the effectiveness and appropriateness of medical care, considerable scientific evidence exists in many areas. Major national organizations, both governmental and professional, are moving to translate existing scientific evidence into practice policies and guidelines. The challenge for clinical leaders is to *implement* existing knowledge into the day-to-day practice of medicine, and guidelines are proving to be a helpful tool. Perhaps a less glamorous undertaking—translating existing scientific knowledge into measurable routine practice patterns—is a major frontier for the 1990s. Finding the practical solutions that take what is known about optimal practices and achieving measurable conformance to evidence-based practice guidelines and competitive prices will separate winners and losers in many health care markets.

There is substantial evidence that guidelines of all types can help practitioners succeed in improving quality of care and efficiency (Kelly and Toepp, 1992). Implementing guidelines and pathways can reduce costs and clinical complications. Guidelines have been used successfully to decrease cesarean section rates without increase in maternal or fetal morbidity. They have supported anesthesiologists in reducing hypoxic injuries and improved the appropriate utilization of coronary care units. Pathways, tools that map the daily or weekly care to patients, can clarify where scientific evidence or professional consensus exists concerning optimal clinical practice and where it is lacking (Grilli and Lomas, 1994). Alternatively, decision-making algorithms can reduce variation for key decision points in a care process (Schriefer, 1994). These tools can be used effectively in combination by applying paths to more routine sequences of process steps and algorithms to help make diagnosis and treatment decisions.

By implementing guidelines that reflect current scientific evidence, quality planning projects can support clinicians in their efforts on behalf of their patients. If used properly, they can create a supportive teamwork environment among physicians and between specialties. Guidelines and pathways can serve as the basis for communication, measurement, and decision support aids. Guidelines have been shown to be an effective tool, when used in conjunction with feedback, decision supports, and other quality improvement tools (Lomas, 1989; Mugford, Banfield, and O'Hanlon, 1991; Weingarten and Ellrodt, 1992). They have not proved effective as directives, in the absence of feedback, reminders, or decision aids (Armstrong, 1994; Kosecoff and others, 1987; Lomas, 1989).

Guidelines are only a tool. Like all tools, they are a means to an end, not the end in and of itself. "Clinical practice guidelines can improve health care outcomes, but they are only as effective as their implementation," wrote Matthew Handley, director of medical education for the Group Health Cooperative of Seattle (Handley, Stuart, and Kirz, 1994, p. 82). Guidelines can be useful in some, but not all, circumstances. Used incorrectly, they can become a tool for one professional group to "manage" another. They can become a source of unnecessary conflict and inflame undue professional resistance to quality management. They can stifle innovation and foster rigidity.

They can also waste precious quality management resources without achieving measurable improvement in outcomes or efficiency. Appropriate use of guidelines, in conjunction with measurement, feedback, and experimentation, can be effective in improving cost efficiency and results of care.

## When Are Guidelines the Right Tool?

Guideline tools are most effective when they are designed and implemented following the basic quality planning principles. The key is making wise decisions about when and how to use guidelines and choosing the right type of guideline tool for the diagnosis or process selected for redesign.

There are a variety of tools available. A guideline applies "if the outcomes of the intervention are well enough understood to permit decisions about its proper use, and if it is preferred . . . by an appreciable but not unanimous majority" (Eddy, 1992, p. 9). Types of guidelines useful for managing outcomes and variation in practice include pathways, protocols, algorithms, precertification, utilization review, reimbursement, and credentialing. Each is a tool to foster consistency and correctness of process of care—the right way to practice. They should be designed to combine scientific evidence with practitioners' experience and opinions to document and specify the intended practice within a group, medical staff, or institution. There should be congruity between all guidelines within a health care system. For example, in a managed-care organization, guidelines for reimbursement, precertification, and clinical practice should be consistent to be effective among practitioners. Consistency of guidelines can be a test of credibility among providers.

Choosing the correct tool depends on the problem to be solved. Pathways and protocols are guidelines for care that are related to time, most often applied to inpatient care but relevant to ambulatory care as well. They represent the ideal sequence and timing of events. A good pathway targets expected outcomes of each time period and allows for charting of intermediate clinical outcomes and variances from the pathway. Standing orders and protocols are variations on a pathway. Standing orders are a tool to address one point in time, such as admission for a particular diagnosis or procedure. Protocols are very similar to pathways, but as the name implies, there is intent to evaluate the effectiveness of the care process as well as the outcomes. The name sounds less proscriptive, which has advantages. Maintaining an openness to improve pathways interactively is an important feature of successful pathway implementation.

Pathways apply to a well-defined cohort of comparable patients whose care is appropriately defined by the pathway. They may apply to a diagnostic related group (DRG); a subset of DRGs, such as a grouping of International Classification of Disease, Version 9, codes (ICD-9 codes); or a grouping of DRGs. (Both of these grouping methods were designed for purposes other than quality management.) There are a number of classification systems in use for payment purposes that can be used, with some effort, to identify a clinically meaningful cohort of patients whose outcomes can be compared.

The most common successes using pathways have been with uncomplicated procedures such as cesarean section, hip replacement, and coronary artery bypass (see Exhibit 5.1). These situations lend themselves to pathways because the pathway is applied *after* the decision to perform the procedure. There is often consensus

Exhibit 5.1. Sample Pathway: Coronary Artery Bypass Surgery.

|  | Pre-Op Day | Op Day (presurgery) | Op Day (postsurgery) | Post-Op (day 1) |
|---|---|---|---|---|
| Tests |  |  |  |  |
| Treatments |  |  |  |  |
| Medications |  |  |  |  |
| Education |  |  |  |  |

among practitioners caring for these cohorts of patients about the way their care should be managed throughout their episode of care. Some organizations find pathways helpful for chronic physiologic conditions that require managing several physiologic parameters simultaneously, such as congestive heart failure, diabetes, and ventilator weaning. This application tends to be problematic.

For more acute diagnoses such as pneumonia or myocardial infarction, pathways appear to be less useful. For example, the critical steps in caring for a patient with pneumonia occur in the first few hours of care. The key steps in the process include collecting specimens for culture swiftly and accurately, followed by initiation of appropriate antibiotic therapy. There are multiple decisions to make, based on clinical information. A similar situation exists for the management of myocardial infarction, acute asthma, or pos-operative arrhythmia. In these situations, a decision-making algorithm that supports swift, correct diagnosis will contribute to achieving optimal patient outcomes.

### Juran and Practice Guidelines

In the Juran Trilogy, quality planning is the work of designing and implementing the best possible care processes. The quality planning process is a structured participatory approach to determining patients' and purchasers' (customer) needs, combining customer needs with scientific knowledge in the design of care processes, identifying what clinicians and other staff (suppliers) need in order to provide care consistent with guidelines, and successfully implementing new processes. Quality planning includes such activities as clinical guideline development and implementation. It also applies to designing delivery processes, such as emergency room triage, post-discharge home care, abnormal laboratory test follow-up, and any other cross-functional processes that affect patient outcomes. Quality planning or guideline teams should be chartered and followed by a steering group or quality council, just like teams using other approaches and tools to improve quality to patients.

Quality planning is a systematic way to achieve the following tasks:

- Establish a project with clear goals and a team to lead the work

- Determine customer needs and expectations

- Design clinical care that meets patients' needs based on the scientific evidence

- Design administrative processes that support clinical decision making specified by guidelines

- Use and evaluate care paths and guidelines

## Quality Planning: Case Studies

Increasingly, there are public domain guidelines available for use. Resources such as the AMA *Directory of Clinical Parameters* and the *Agency for Health Care Policy and Research* are focused on compiling listings of available guidelines. Another source is the quality and outcomes trade literature, which tends to feature cases from organizations around the country (see the Recommended Reading section at the back of the book). Often organizations are willing to share their guidelines free or at cost. There are also commercially available guidelines.

What about the quality of the final results? How satisfied will patients and physicians be with the care and outcomes? Quality planning is a set of activities designed to optimize the quality of care delivered relative to patient and purchaser needs as well as professional standards of practice.

### Case Example: Scripps Health System, La Jolla, California

This system developed a program to improve the efficiency of managing cardiac surgery patients and improve clinical and satisfaction outcome measures. Clinicians, working in a multidisciplinary team, specified the process of managing cardiac surgery patients. They translated these process specifications into written, step-by-step plans (one for physicians and one for patients) used to document and monitor treatment and outcomes. Within seven months of implementing the new process, there was a 22 percent decrease in length of stay, 12.3 percent decrease in charges, and a 40 to 50 percent decline in physician and nurse paperwork time. Patient satisfaction improved simultaneously, in part due to the project and its emphasis on patient information and individualized care (Andersson, 1993).

### Case Example: Group Health Cooperative (GHC), Puget Sound, Washington

GHC formed a multidisciplinary committee on prevention whose purpose is to define and implement prevention guidelines. Since 1978, the committee has addressed over fifty major preventive care issues and laid the foundation for new medical practice guidelines. Some guidelines suggested increased services (mammography); others led to the discontinuation of nonefficacious practices (screening chest X-rays) and reduced resource use. Overall, guideline development, implementation, measurement, and feedback led to a reduction in variation in prevention practices for GHC (Davis, 1991).

### Case Example: Kaiser Permanente, Milpitas, California

With asthma morbidity and mortality on the rise, many managed-care organizations are implementing nationally endorsed practice guidelines to reduce morbidity and hospitalizations (Lanman, 1994). The pediatrics department at this clinic implemented practice changes and reduced hospital admissions for asthma with three interventions. They profiled physician admission rates and feedback with comparisons within their peer group, sponsored a survey of pediatrician asthma practice patterns and feedback about variation in practice style, and promoted the National Asthma Education Project guideline, particularly use of peak flow meters and inhaled steroids. They found striking variation in practices and admission rates, including a fourfold variation in admission rates for children aged one to fourteen, despite an overall average well below the national average. With continued measurement, feedback, dialogue, and issuing their own version summary of the national guideline, admission rates appeared to decline significantly.

## Quality Planning: A Structured Process

Quality planning is a structured, participatory approach to designing new or redesigning existing clinical services. It provides a forum for clinicians and other professionals to identify where there is evidence and consensus concerning best practices.

For successful guideline projects, identifying the evidence for best practice is just the beginning. The harder and more important stage is implementation—ensuring that all patients with comparable disease receive care consistent with the best demonstrated practice. Patients and payers are intolerant of variation in practice that cannot be justified on the basis of outcomes or efficiency. They expect the medical profession to achieve consensus and to use research methods to identify which treatment strategies work best and most cost effectively. Patients, particularly patients in organized delivery systems, want to have confidence that regardless of which clinician they see, their care will be the same as it would have been had they seen their own personal doctor.

A planning team, like most clinical practice teams, should be cross-functional, with representatives from all relevant specialties and professional groups. It should include seven to ten individuals charged with representing their constituency. Planning teams use tools and a step-wise process to identify patient needs, design clinical care, design the delivery process, and use and evaluate the new care process (see Figure 5.1).

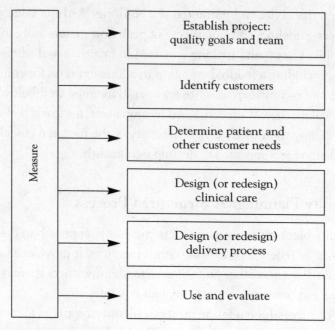

Figure 5.1. Quality Planning.

## Establishing a Goal

Quality planning teams should be chartered by a steering group or quality council, just like improvement teams and measurement teams, as part of a comprehensive strategy for quality. Before beginning work, a team needs clearly defined goals and a timetable for accomplishing its charter. All project teams are expensive, regardless of the tools and techniques they use to create higher quality. They should add measurable value to the organization and demonstrate visible impact on patients within three to six months. This is crucial—practitioners have limited time and organizations have limited resources. Visible, rapid impact needs to drive the design of all projects.

The first step is to define a charter for the project (see Exhibit 5.2) based on the following questions:

What clinical care process is the team going to design?

Exhibit 5.2.  Sample Project Charter.
- Design prenatal and early life care to high-risk mothers and babies.

- Increase high-risk mother participation in program by 20 percent.

- Reduce the NICU costs by 20 percent.

- Reduce the LBWB rate by 10 percent.

- Increase MD satisfaction with support program by 25 percent.

Which patient populations does this affect?

What evidence (data) exists to support working on this process?

What quality or cost problem must be solved?

What are the health status and clinical outcome objectives, cost objectives, patient satisfaction objectives, and benchmarks?

What are the boundaries of the process and project?

What is the expected outcome of this project team? When?

### Identifying Customers and Their Needs

The team identifies the customer groups who depend on the care selected for design. Obviously, there is some form of care already in place so that in essence, all clinical care planning projects are actually redesigning an existing process. There are several external customer groups—different patient populations and purchasers. There are also internal customer groups or suppliers—clinicians, their office staffs, and various vendors involved in the care to the patients.

### Determining Patient and Other Customer Needs

Next, it is essential to analyze customer needs, both stated and real needs. Customers will identify many of their needs clearly and explicitly. In other cases, stated needs actually reflect some other more basic need (Juran, 1989). Uncovering the real need behind the stated need provides a major advantage in designing care processes that lead to patient loyalty as well as satisfaction.

Determining patient needs can follow a three-phase process:

- *Analyze* historic patterns.

- *Ask* the patients what they need and want, using focus groups, surveys, and interviews.

- *Collect feedback* on their satisfaction or dissatisfaction.

If the planning team fully understands patients' needs, it is more likely to design a process patients will comply with and recommend to other patients. Unstated or cultural needs are often the basis for creating features with attractive quality.

For example, a quality planning team was chartered to reduce the asthma admission rate for children. They made assumptions about parents who seek after-hours urgent care and tried to redesign the process to ensure that these families saw practitioners during the day on a regular basis for maintenance visits. The intervention failed: the hospital admission rate remained high and mothers generally canceled their follow-up ambulatory visits. The team had failed to realize that the population they needed to reach was working mothers who could not afford to take time off from work for daytime visits. They needed a process that provided after-hours visits for maintenance care of their asthmatic children. Without this understanding of customer needs, the team designed the wrong process change and did not improve the asthma admission rate.

### Customer Needs Analysis Techniques

Most of the techniques for determining customer needs derive from market research. They consist of methods to elicit needs of individuals and patient cohorts.

One popular method is focus groups, which allow for open-ended and targeted questioning. For example, University of Wisconsin used focus groups to learn about breast cancer patients' and their families' needs during treatment (Gustafson, Taylor, Thompson, and Chesney, 1993). In a focus group, participants build on one another's comments and increase the volume and creativity of ideas. However, sometimes they intimidate minority viewpoints from being expressed.

Two other familiar techniques are surveys and interviews. Surveys are very useful when reliability between respondents is important. They have the shortcoming of leaving open the issue of who and why some people are nonrespondents. Interviews can be structured or informal, depending on the objective. Structured interviews yield information very similar to surveys. Open-ended interviews involve asking questions such as "What didn't you like about your experience in our hospital?" or "What could we have done to make you less anxious during your illness?" These can yield insightful observations and creative ideas.

Complaints are another important source of information about patients. As a general management practice, all complaints and grievances should be reviewed periodically. They can provide insight into needs that are not being met in specific processes. However, the absence of complaints about a particular process cannot be taken to mean patients are delighted with their care and loyal to their caregivers. It is easy to encourage or discourage complaints.

### Keeping Track of Needs

Quality planning often generates a great deal of information. It is helpful to organize all this information in a systematic format. Exhibit 5.3 displays one of several types of spreadsheets that has been helpful to quality planning teams in organizing their information on customer needs.

Not only can a spreadsheet be used to keep track of different patient cohorts and their needs, but it can be used to balance

Exhibit 5.3. Displaying Customer Research.

| Customer | Need | Details | Supplier translation | Outcomes measures |
|---|---|---|---|---|
| 15-yo $G_2Ab_2P_0$ smoker, alcoholic | Healthy baby | No specialized care | No NICU care | LOS |
| | | | | Weight > 1,500 gr |
| | | | | Gestation > 34 wk |
| | | | | Apgar > 7 |
| | | No preventable disabilities | Normal language development | Developmental scores |
| | | | Normal motor skills development | Motor skills scores |
| | | Information about preterm labor | Age, appropriate education | Seek treatment for correct indications |

purchasers' and managed-care organizations' needs as well. In competitive markets, for example, hospitals have to balance various patient populations along with different health plans, each with differing needs and priorities. Quality planning teams must be able to make careful judgments about how to respond to conflicting and complex expectations. Juran (1989) addressed several types of spreadsheets to display and analyze customer needs.

## Designing Clinical Care

To suggest that planning teams design clinical care is misleading. Care is delivered to patients every day. However, given the presence of substantial variation, limited supporting scientific evidence, and lack of consensus among clinicians, it appears that much of clinical practice is idiosyncratic. A practice guideline or pathway is a tool to clarify and illuminate variation, to foster awareness of the impact of different clinical decisions, and to encourage reduction in variation if it adds no demonstrable value to patients.

There are several approaches currently in use for developing evidence-based and consensus guidelines. The focus of national guidelines published by medical specialty societies and the Agency for Health Care Policy and Research has been on broad *evidence-based* policies related to the appropriate indications for technology and procedure use—an important step. These guidelines can address such issues as whether, for example, cystoscopy has been shown to improve the diagnostic accuracy and outcomes for patients with benign prostatic hypertrophy considering transurethral prostatectomy. They often are too high-level, however, to meet the day-to-day needs of clinicians and their patients. Pathway development is more of an operational on-line endeavor, and the successful examples are found in quality management and nursing literature (Coffey and others, 1992; Zander, 1991).

The experience with *consensus-based* guidelines is problematic in a different way. It has been shown that different groups of clinicians will develop different guidelines, particularly when the representation of specialties varies (Eddy and Billings, 1988). Because of these experiences, there is intensified pressure to document the scientific evidence justifying particular care processes.

Within organizations using guidelines as a tool to manage quality, both evidence and consensus are incorporated into guidelines and pathways (Schriefer, 1994). Benchmark organizations using guidelines and pathways in clinical practice commonly use five basic steps to develop a pathway or algorithm. (For more detail, Hofmann's excellent generic development process, published in 1993, goes stepwise through from topic to critical path, using both scientific evidence from the literature and consensus from practitioners.)

## Model for Clinical Care Design

1. Describe current clinical process.

2. Compare with literature and colleagues.

3. Identify "best" practice, if known.

4. Build consensus for best practice.

5. Design for patient and other customer needs.

## Understanding Current Clinical Process

Begin by describing the current clinical process, collecting and analyzing existing data to demonstrate variation in practice patterns for comparable patients. For example, describe the range in drug regimens for comparable patients with chronic asthma and the use of inhaled steroids or home nebulizer treatments. Similarly, describe the variability in timing to initiation of antibiotics or requests for infectious disease consultation for pneumonia patients. When high rates of variability are found and inexplicable, clinicians are typically open to looking at how their practices compare to published studies or colleagues in comparable settings.

This step should be done without significant data collection. Use existing administrative or quality assurance data, a quick survey to practitioners about their beliefs, or simple chart review (Lanman, 1994). It is not necessary or helpful to create a major data collection and data base to get an adequate understanding of current practices. Some teams get stuck at this point, assuming that a large, risk-adjusted data collection is needed before they can improve care to patients. It is important to steer them out of this off-line mindset and onto a more practical, on-line approach to fixing obvious quality deficiencies and making rapid process enhancements.

## Comparisons with Evidence and Peers and Identifying Best Practice

Comparing documented process of care patterns or outcomes to those of other similar organizations is typically provocative, usually in a positive manner. Raising questions and answering them with information about local and regional practice patterns is a constructive approach, particularly if done in a spirit of openness about the best method of practice. Sometimes it is possible to identify best practice, based on scientific literature; at other times, the evidence is inadequate. It is critical to strike a balance between what can be justified by scientific evidence and therefore written into a guideline, and what is clinician experience or opinion and therefore unproven.

## Building Consensus for Best Practice

When best practices are clearly defined by the scientific evidence, using opinion leaders to encourage adherence to a guideline or care path is appropriate. When evidence-justified best practices are unavailable, the next step is to motivate practitioners to practice according to operational research protocols and thereby allow for the discovery of new knowledge about best practices.

Brent James, executive director of Intermountain Health Care's Center for Health Care Delivery Research and a national leader in clinical quality management, is well known for asking clinicians to practice according to research protocols, to allow for the evaluation of practice patterns: "It's more important that you do it the *same* than that you do it 'right.'" This does not necessarily mean that all clinicians must follow some cookbook approach to their patients. Quite to the contrary, it means health care organizations will assume more responsibility in evaluating the effectiveness of their practices.

## Innovation in Design

As a team plans care that represents the best in scientific application and is the most responsive to customer needs, it may have the opportunity to introduce significant innovations. Planners should always pause in their analysis, evaluate all they have learned, and ask, "Are there radically different designs that could produce quantum leaps in outcomes or satisfaction?" Stimulating planners to think creatively will often pay handsome dividends. Naturally, most innovations will require testing before being implemented to determine if they will have the desired effect on patient satisfaction, outcome, or cost.

## Designing the Delivery Process

With any guideline or path, the design team needs to address the readiness of practitioners and the delivery system to implement the guideline. To foster practice pattern change to comply with this guideline, as with any guideline, there are three issues that must be addressed:

1. Practitioner education and buy-in

2. Operational process capacity

3. Patients' expectations and needs

Guidelines are a translation of scientific evidence into a specification of process—a statement of intention within an organized delivery system. The issue of practitioner communication and education requires more than an "FYI." Resistance mounts quickly without systematic attention to diversity of opinions, variable knowledge and skill sets, and system supports to practitioners (Fink, Kosecoff, Chassin, and Brook, 1984; Schoenbaum and Gottlieb, 1990).

*Model for Administrative Process Design*

1. Assess administrative system capacity and interdependencies.

2. Conduct failure analysis.

3. Use and evaluate.

4. Demonstrate collaboration and leadership.

If such a process specification is to be implemented by practitioners, there must be capacity in a variety of administrative processes (Barton and Schoenbaum, 1990). Consider a health plan that adopts a guideline stating that all women evaluated by an internist for a breast lump should be seen by a surgeon within one week (Gottlieb, Sokol, Murray, and Schoenbaum, 1992). While there is limited scientific evidence to suggest such a guideline is necessary, this health plan chose to establish this guideline because its evidence on member satisfaction suggested that women with breast lumps tolerate only a two-week wait for surgical consultation. Beyond two weeks, their confidence in the health plan drops and their anxiety level rises.

Assuming there is general agreement among practitioners that this guideline is worth implementing, there are the practical realities of systems and processes and their inherent capacity. There may be limitations in the capacity of processes, such as appointment scheduling, surgical ambulatory visits, and mammography, that make implementing this guideline impossible.

Two tools are often used by design teams to address these issues and prevent problems and failures. One tool useful at this stage is the cause-and-effect diagram or Ishikawa diagram (Ishikawa, 1982). Consider a prenatal care program for high-risk pregnancies. There are a number of potential sources of program failure that will have greater or lesser impact on the outcome of interest: low-birth-weight rates. It is important for quality planning teams to analyze whether the interventions in the process of care they propose are feasible and have a high probability of achieving the desired result. Using a cause-and-effect diagram (Figure 5.2), a cross-functional planning team can address where the proposed process changes may fail to give women at risk for preterm labor what they need. They can identify where obstetricians and case managers need to ensure thorough coordination and communication.

Another useful tool is the "failure mode and effect analysis" (see Exhibit 5.4). This matrix tool helps the design team systematically evaluate the possible causes of failure and plan for alternative strategies to prevent them (Juran and Gryna, 1988, pp. 13-28–13-36).

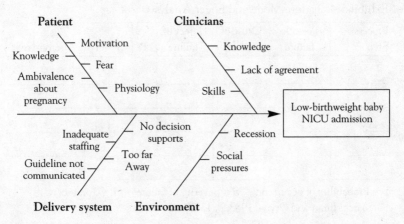

Figure 5.2.  Sample Cause-and-Effect Diagram: High-Risk Pregnancy.

## Use and Evaluation

Guidelines, algorithms, and pathways are critical components of the quality management program within a clinical organization. Together with feedback and reminders, they are important tools to use in managing clinical quality. Like all tools, they are a means to an end. Debating the virtues of various quality tools would be like carpenters debating hammers and wrenches. The only meaningful question is, What are you trying to accomplish and which tools do you need to use?

Guidelines must be viewed as part of the clinical support services provided to clinicians to support them in caring for patients. If they are seen as a dictate issued from management, there will be resistance and loss of morale. If they are presented as part of a comprehensive program to identify and support best practices, clinicians will recognize the value of guidelines and make creative contributions that lead to breakthroughs in organizational performance.

## Keys to Implementation

Several organizations and academic researchers have reviewed the practical lessons associated with successful guideline implementation

Exhibit 5.4. Failure Mode and Effect Analysis.

| Process Step | Possible failure | Cause of failure | Effect of failure | P | S | T | Alternatives |
|---|---|---|---|---|---|---|---|
|  |  |  |  |  |  |  |  |
|  |  |  |  |  |  |  |  |
|  |  |  |  |  |  |  |  |
|  |  |  |  |  |  |  |  |
|  |  |  |  |  |  |  |  |

P = Probability of occurrence   S = Severity of failure   T = Total score
  *Source:* Juran and Gryna, 1988, p. 13-28.

(Handley, Stuart, and Kirz, 1994; Lomas and Haynes, 1988; Lomas and others, 1991; Schriefer, 1994; Weingarten and Ellrodt, 1992). Guidelines have been in use widely for a number of years, and there are some clear keys to their successful implementation. The most basic lesson is that implementation means much more than distributing a notebook for practitioners to read. Many organizations have found that published guidelines often sit on clinicians' shelves, ignored like other edicts from management. Successful implementation requires multifaceted interventions. The work of quality planning teams is not complete until measurable impact is achieved.

## Leadership Style

For organizations using guidelines and paths, it is important to define a leadership style that fosters collaboration with clinicians. If they are offered with an open style and as part of a comprehensive approach to discovering and replicating best practices, some of the natural resistance from clinicians can be minimized. When practitioners perceive a patronizing attitude from clinical leaders, they tend to dismiss guidelines.

Clinicians are particularly attentive to the messenger. If the guideline supporters are opinion leaders in the care to the diagnostic group addressed in the guideline, peers are far more likely to listen. This means physicians involved in promoting guidelines should identify those opinion leaders and put them in the role of promoting the guidelines (schedule them to speak at staff meetings, department meetings, grand rounds). Academic detailing, a variant on drug company detailing, using physician opinion leaders, is particularly effective.

## Proving the Need

Clinicians need data to prove that they need to change. They need direct motivation based on their ability to compete for patients or risks to the patients they care for. The proof must be compelling, immediate, and data driven. Without a proof of the need to change and a connection to the guideline proposed, clinicians may dismiss the guideline as academic or irrelevant to them.

## Clear Objectives

Objectives of any management tool intended to change practice patterns must be focused and clear. It must be obvious what the objective is and how it is related to the need to change. General goodness of practice is not specific enough to capture the attention of busy clinicians. It is also important that the patient cohort addressed by the guideline be clear and targeted and that the number of changes introduced at any one time be limited.

## Combining National Guidelines with Local Style

Designing guidelines can be costly. It is important to draw on existing guidelines, algorithms, and pathways whenever possible. For many organizations, drawing on nationally known sources helps to lend credibility to the guidelines. However, there must always be an opportunity for clinicians to review and modify guidelines before implementation. Never attempt to implement a "black box." The logic and criteria of a guideline must be open and available prospectively to practitioners. Typically, when the basis for a guideline is defensible scientific evidence, this step is more about understanding a guideline than it is about changing it.

## Flexibility

Treat guideline implementation as an iterative process. Make clear to practitioners that they will change and enhance the guideline over time as they learn more about the variation in their patient-care processes. Make following the guideline voluntary whenever appropriate. As practitioners use the guideline over time, measure the acceptance rate and report on the general practitioner acceptance of the guideline. This approach fosters an atmosphere of continuous improvement and innovation.

## Multiple Process Interventions

Successful projects use a number of interventions to change the process. Rarely is one silver bullet discovered. To be successful, guidelines need to be combined with education, measurement and feedback, decision supports and reminders, and patient education and incentives.

## Measurement and Feedback

Typically, successful projects combine feedback with guideline development and implementation. The keys here are to tailor the feedback to the practice issues addressed by the guideline and to make the feedback as current as possible. Clinicians are naturally more responsive to data they request because they are invested in the process of changing practice patterns. Unsolicited feedback results in less impact than feedback that practitioners actively seek out.

It helps to use practitioners' input into the design of feedback reports. At Blue Cross and Blue Shield of Massachusetts, practitioners were provided multiple opportunities to provide customer input during the design phase of feedback reports. The input led to major enhancements in the design of the reports as well as greater interest in the reports once they were made available.

## Clinical Decision Supports and Reminders

Job aids to support good practice are not new to medicine. The asterisk beside an abnormal laboratory value is an aid. Computerized reminders have proved very useful (Tierney, Hui, and McDonald, 1986). Simple tools such as pocket formularies and laminated cards can be very effective. The key is to identify whether the process deficiency needing improvement may be due to the challenge of keeping all necessary information handy at the time of patient encounters. Rather than cookbook medicine, well-positioned reminders can be a welcome support by practitioners.

### Interventions Involving Patients

For practices that are in large part responsive to patient demand, interventions directed at demand reduction or change in patient attitude may be the most effective. For example, consider the change in smoking behaviors witnessed over the past decade. While physicians have been shown to affect patient smoking behavior, the lay press and public policy have played an even greater role in reducing smoking among some populations.

A major issue for managed-care organizations is to reduce demand for unnecessary office visits. For staff-model or capitated HMOs, there is a need to manage patient demand for care when self-care or simple telephone advice is more appropriate. In these situations, focusing on patient demand will have higher yield than guidelines or feedback to practitioners who want to satisfy their patients.

Another example is found in projects to reduce inappropriately high cesarean section rates. While there is a need for practitioner and delivery system changes, patient and family attitudes about vaginal birth after cesarean section are also important. By reducing patient demand for cesarean deliveries, practitioners are more likely to succeed in their efforts to reduce their rates.

### Administrative and System Revisions

Physicians do not always control the process of care. While they may intend for their patients to receive appropriate care in a timely manner, they function within delivery systems that cannot always implement physician orders as written. The best guideline in the profession can lie dormant if administrative policies and procedures obstruct their implementation. Often successful implementation of a guideline requires revising an administrative process.

## Conclusion

Successful use of guidelines in quality management programs requires understanding how and when to use the tools. It is like diagnosing and treating an illness. There are multiple diagnostic tests and treatments required for different patients at different stages of their disease. There is no one silver bullet for most illnesses. Different problems are solved using different tools. The key is to use the right tool in the right way within an overall strategy to achieve a successful outcome.

# 6

# Practice and
# Outcomes Improvement

For a health care organization to be competitive, clinicians must have a game plan to address measurement, feedback, and improvement. Chapter Four describes techniques and tools for measuring practice patterns and outcomes and reducing unintended variation (quality control). Chapter Five describes how and when to develop practice guidelines as a means to create new practice patterns and strategies for patient-focused care. It introduces design and planning techniques for achieving innovations in patient-focused care and outcomes (quality planning). This chapter describes practice and outcomes improvement, the basic approach to improving existing clinical processes (quality improvement).

Quality control activities rely on tools and methods of measuring performance, feeding back information about performance, and decreasing unnecessary practice variation. Quality planning projects address care processes that are too dysfunctional to simply improve. Quality planning teams set aside the existing process and design innovative care processes that will produce significantly better patient outcomes and satisfaction. Another term for this type of design project is *reengineering*. The approach most useful and most relevant to clinical care is quality improvement. It is a simple, relatively quick approach to diagnosing what can be changed in clinical care to result in better patient outcomes and satisfaction. Because there is significant waste in health care today, often quality improvement projects reduce cost as well. Quality planning projects can require several months and substantial resources to complete. Quality improvement projects, by contrast, tackle simpler problems with less time and resources.

Clinical process improvement in a hospital, group practice, or HMO takes place on a project-by-project basis. It requires analyzing existing care processes, identifying root cause or causes of cost and quality problems, and it identifies changes in clinical and administrative practices to ensure better performance. Improvement teams use specific tools and techniques to diagnose problems, identify root causes of current deficiencies, and change practice patterns and administrative procedures (Goal/QPC, 1988; Juran Institute, 1993a; Plsek, 1989; Scholtes and others, 1988).

The quality improvement model is akin to clinical practice and the scientific method. It relies on the basic concepts of hypothesis testing and applies these techniques to practice patterns and outcomes. There are many processes in hospital and ambulatory settings that do not meet the expectations of patients, clinicians, and payers. Chronic problems are excellent topics for successful quality improvement projects.

While quality improvement projects are grounded in the scientific method, they are fundamentally different from classical research on health care effectiveness. They are on-line projects that result in improvement in the patient care within an organization, but they lack the rigor of a research project designed to prove causality or efficacy of an intervention. They also require much less resource to implement. Results should be measurable within a few months. They may not yield generalized lessons or new knowledge about clinical care, although they always yield better outcomes for patients of that particular hospital or group practice. By doing so, they are critical to continuous improvement within an organization and economic survival long term. Today, demonstrating improvement is not only required for accreditation by the Joint Commission on Accreditation of Healthcare Organizations and the National

Committee on Quality Assurance, it is increasingly required by purchasers to maintain managed-care and employer contracts.

## Case Study: Reduction in Cesarean Section Rates

Many hospitals are pressured by managed care or purchasers to reduce their cesarean section rate. While the correct rate is unknown, there is widespread opinion and evidence to suggest that rates of 20 to 30 percent or higher are excessive. Some hospitals successfully lower their rates using measurement and feedback of physician-specific rates to obstetricians. At other hospitals, quality improvement teams analyze root causes and identify process interventions to reduce their rates even further.

At a community hospital the section rate was in the 20 to 25 percent range in the late 1980s, despite tracking and reporting the rates. A cross-functional team representing obstetrics, obstetrical nursing, anesthesia, and administration analyzed data existing in the obstetrical log. They discovered that repeat C-sections were particularly common and developed theories of cause for repeats. They collecting data from patients and confirmed that some beliefs and assumptions were common, such as "once a section, always a section." All the data were plotted on a cause-and-effect diagram (Figure 6.1).

The first remedy the team evaluated and implemented was an adjunct birthing class for expectant mothers who previously delivered by section. The team evaluated the impact of the intervention by tracking the percentage of these women who attempted labor. The attempt rate went from 77 to 92 percent. The overall section rate dropped from 22 to 17 percent during this time of this educational intervention.

The second most common cause of reluctance to attempt vaginal birth after cesarean (VBAC) was the attitude of the expectant grandmothers. Often they had given birth during the 1950s when VBACs were rare, and they strongly resisted the idea. The next

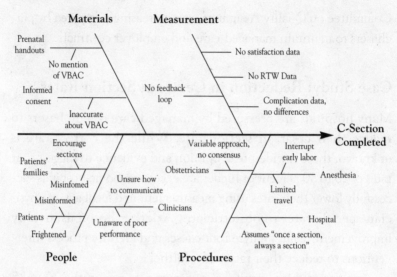

Figure 6.1. High-C-Section-Rate Cause-and-Effect Diagram.

intervention was to invite the grandmothers to the birth education classes and to inform them on the safety and benefits of VBACs. This intervention brought the section rate down to between 10 and 14 percent. The team also found that by plotting their simple data on a scatter plot (Figure 6.2), they could see that the maximum optimal trial of labor was up to about twelve to sixteen hours. After that, the VBAC success rate dropped off. This helped them in their management of patients in labor.

This project was not designed to prove the effectiveness of birth education on VBAC. The goal of the project was not to publish an academic article. That would require more statistical rigor and expense. The goal was to successfully lower the C-section rate without patient complications—and it was achieved.

## Case Study: Chest Pain Management

The managed-care market in Atlanta is competitive. Hospitals must demonstrate they can improve quality and lower cost to maintain contracts. PruCare, which accounts for about 20 percent of the

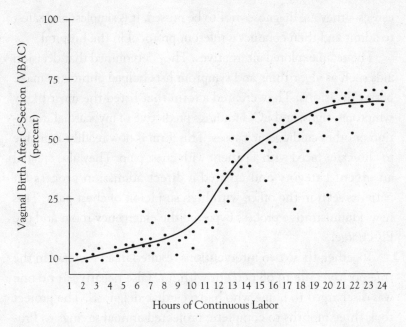

Figure 6.2.  Cesarean Section Labor Scatter Diagram.

business at West Paces Ferry Hospital, targeted care to patients with cardiac disease for improvement goals at its hospitals. It set an expectation to reduce unnecessary admissions to the hospital for noncardiogenic chest pain (Caldwell, 1994).

West Paces chartered an improvement team with representation from internal medicine, emergency medicine, cardiology, family practice, nursing, and administration. There were hospital and managed-care team members. The team reviewed eighty charts of PruCare patients admitted with chest pain. Of the eighty, twenty-two were discharged with a cardiac diagnosis, producing a "true positive" admission rate for cardiogenic causes of about 28 percent. The clinical team brainstormed possible causes of the low true positive rate and tested their theories. They determined that clinicians in an emergency room are under pressure to move patients through and either admit them or discharge them. With chest pain, clinicians as well as patients have substantial anxiety about cardiogenic causes—they are diagnoses not to be missed. It is simplest and safest to admit and then conduct a rule-out protocol in the hospital.

The team explored alternatives. They determined that decision aids such as algorithms and symptom lists helped clinicians make better decisions. They created a form that listed the most likely symptoms, signs, and ECG findings predictive of myocardial infarction or other cardiogenic causes. This form is now readily available to clinicians faced with a patient with chest pain. They also created an urgent category and created a direct admission process for patients seen in the office with high suspicion of chest pain. This new administrative process bypassed the emergency room and the ER charge.

Together, these two interventions resulted in an increase in the true positive rate to 68 percent with no "false negatives"; no one was discharged to home who had a cardiac diagnosis. The project took three months to complete; projected annual savings to Pru-Care is $330,000.

## The Six Steps of Quality Improvement

The quality improvement process is identical to clinical medicine—diagnose the cause and then use tested interventions to improve the process. The remainder of the chapter will focus on the six specific steps needed to make improvements. Each step uses tools and scientific evidence. Table 6.1 displays a matrix of the tools and techniques useful at each step.

1. *Identify a project.* Quality within a complex system such as clinical medicine is never improved in a nonspecific way. Improvement will be optimal when it occurs project by project, beginning with the most visible and significant problems.

2. *Establish the project.* The deficiency to be attacked must be clearly specified and the expected improvement defined in

measurable terms. A cross-functional team is assigned to the project and given the time and resources (staff, training, team facilitation, and data) it needs to be successful.

3. *Diagnose the cause.* The team uses the scientific method and basic diagnostic tools (flow diagrams, simple data collection, cause-and-effect diagrams, and so on) to uncover the root causes of deficiencies.

4. *Remedy the cause.* Once the root causes have been clearly identified, an effective process intervention can be designed. The remedy may necessitate enlisting clinician willingness to change their practice patterns or modifying systems within the organization, or both. An effective remedy produces optimal outcomes and results for patients as well as supporting and accommodating needs of clinicians.

5. *Hold the gains.* A quality improvement team's work is not finished until there is a procedure in place to hold the gains. All the work that goes into producing improved results can be lost if there are no effective supports and controls in place.

6. *Replicate results and nominate new projects.* Once a team achieves positive results, there are two final responsibilities: to help others in the organization with similar problems to apply what the team learned from the quality improvement project and to nominate other projects for consideration. When improving any complex process, it is common to uncover other processes and deficiencies that are a chronic source of problems and waste. These should be nominated for other teams to work on.

Each of the six quality improvement steps encompasses several activities. Separating the work into six large steps helps organize and focus the project, but there is no special magic to six steps. The ten-step model from the Joint Commission of Accreditation of Healthcare Organizations and Focus-Plan-Do-Check-Act are also options, and many other models exist. Models have their limitations. As

Table 6.1. Quality Tool Applications.

| Quality Tools | 1a. Nominate projects | 1b. Evaluate projects | 1c. Select a project | 1d. Ask: Is it quality improvement? | 2a. Prepare a mission statement | 2b. Select a team | 2c. Verify the mission | 3a. Analyze the symptoms |
|---|---|---|---|---|---|---|---|---|
| Tree diagram | | | | | | | | |
| Stratification | | □ | □ | | □ | | | ■ |
| Selection matrix | | | ■ | | | | | |
| Scatter diagram | | | | X | | | | |
| Planning network | | | | | | | | |
| Planning matrix | | | | | | | | |
| Pareto analysis | ■ | ■ | ■ | | □ | | | ■ |
| Histogram | | | | X | | | | □ |
| Graphs and charts | □ | | | | □ | □ | | □ |
| Flow diagram | ■ | □ | | □ | □ | □ | | ■ |
| Data collection | ■ | ■ | ■ | ■ | | □ | | ■ |
| Costs of poor quality | ■ | ■ | ■ | | ■ | □ | | ■ |
| Control spreadsheet | | | | | | | | |
| Control chart | | | | | | | | |
| Cause-and-effect diagram | | X | | X | | | | X |
| Brainstorming | ■ | X | | | | | | X |
| Box plot | | | | X | | | | □ |
| Benefit-cost analysis | | | | | | | | |
| Barriers and aids chart | | | | | | | | |

Quality Improvement Steps and Activities

1. Identify a project
   a. Nominate projects
   b. Evaluate projects
   c. Select a project
   d. Ask: Is it quality improvement?
2. Establish the project
   a. Prepare a mission statement
   b. Select a team
   c. Verify the mission
3. Diagnose the cause
   a. Analyze the symptoms

b. Confirm or modify the mission
c. Formulate theories
d. Test theories
e. Identify root cause(s)
4. Remedy the cause
a. Evaluate alternatives
b. Design remedy
c. Design controls
d. Design for culture
e. Prove effectiveness
f. Implement
5. Hold the gains
a. Design effective quality controls
b. Foolproof the remedy
c. Audit the controls
6. Replicate results and nominate new projects
a. Replicate the project results
b. Nominate new projects

■ Frequently used  □ Occasionally used  × Never used  Rarey used

*Source:* © 1993 Juran Institute.

George Box, one of America's leading quality scientists, once said, "All models are wrong; some models are useful." The quality improvement model presented here is only as useful as the results it helps to achieve. More important, its value is in the manner in which it gets adapted by clinicians using it in creative ways to facilitate improvement in the care to their patients.

## Becoming a World-Class Organization

At this point, you may be wondering, How is this process different from all those ineffectual committees? Quality project teams are different in many respects. One critical difference is that projects are formally chartered and monitored. All too often, committees or task forces are formed to take corrective actions, and they never have a well-defined charter or mission. They are not given appropriate authority and responsibility and do not have the support of their colleagues. They lack a scientific approach to problem solving and rarely use on-line data or experiments. Not surprisingly, committees and task forces rarely produce. If they do achieve some improvement, it is rarely sustained.

Quality improvement projects use systematic methods and techniques, are monitored, and their successes are quantified in terms of their value to patients, clinicians, and purchasers. The results are reported publicly and tracked going forward.

Another common question is, Who identifies the projects? Normally, projects are identified by the cross-functional steering group or quality council that oversees the quality program. Projects chartered by the quality council of a hospital or network quality council identify projects on the basis of potential impact on core processes within the delivery system, performance level, and resource use (volume, patient-care impact, or cost). Projects with systemwide importance require the participation of several departments, units, or specialties.

Successful organizations improve at a tremendous rate. Any organization that survives and thrives over time makes continual adjustments and improvements. Most, however, improve at only the most pedestrian rate. The most important distinguishing characteristic between organizations with a competitive rate of improvement and those with a pedestrian rate of improvement is the number of improvements in a span of time (see Figure 6.3). Also contributing to a rate of change is the selection of the most important improvements to be made and the speed with which they are made. This can only be accomplished when an organization has a clear, widely held vision, an understanding of itself as a system, and a culture and framework that support learning and change.

## Step 1: Identify Quality Improvement Projects

Quality improvement is achieved project by project. It is never improved in a general or undefined way. A quality improvement project is a focused effort by clinicians and others to conduct on-line experiments in their daily practice to find the best processes that achieve optimal outcomes. For example, appropriate clinical quality improvement projects might include:

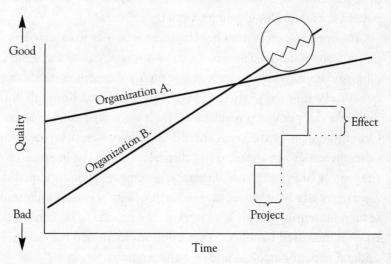

Figure 6.3.  Rate of Improvement.

Reduce the number of postoperative wound infections

Reduce the hours of intubation following cardiac surgery

Increase the percentage of women over fifty receiving annual mammograms

Reduce the time to return to work after hysterectomy

Reduce the number of ER visits among children with asthma

A project that is highly specific, quantifiable, and focused is more likely to succeed. Specificity is important also because it focuses the project. All too often, clinical projects tackle vague goals, such as "improving care to the ventilated patient." Some will be diagnosis-specific, such as reducing work time lost for patients with sciatica; others will be generic care processes, such as reducing nosocomial infections in patients ventilated for five days or more. Projects may address specific deficiencies, such as unacceptably high complication rates, or they may be directed at achieving higher patient functional outcomes or satisfaction with the care they receive. One project, for example, may tackle the rate of adverse drug reactions in the hospital; another may focus on increasing patient confidence in urgent and emergency care.

Time and resources must be allocated for project work. In particular, a team of individuals is required to diagnose causes and design, pilot, and implement solutions. Physician involvement is critical but needs to be tailored to their time constraints. Some hospitals and networks compensate physicians for their work on quality projects. Other members of the team should include representatives from other professions involved.in the clinical process to be improved by the project (nursing, physical therapy, pharmacy, laboratory, quality assurance, administration, and so forth). With a cross-functional team representing people who work in the process to be improved, there is increased likelihood that solutions identified will achieve optimal patient outcomes and cost efficiency.

Let us look at some examples at various levels.

- *Hospital level.* A hospital decides that it could reduce patient complications and increase revenue by reducing the incidence of adverse drug reactions among surgery patients. A team to address this problem would include internal medicine, surgery, nursing, and pharmacy representation.

- *Departmental level.* Pediatricians in an HMO decide to reduce the admission rate for children with asthma. The departmental steering group establishes this as a quality goal and charters a team to improve the ambulatory care process. The team would include pediatricians, nurses, and health educators.

- *Group practice level.* A group practice decides to increase the proportion of patients receiving their abnormal lab results in twenty-four hours and their normal lab results within ten days of their visits. Practice administrators set a goal and charter a team to reduce the time to patient receipt of test results.

The bottom line is that quality is rarely improved by sending memos or writing policies. It is never improved by taking a general approach. An organization enhances quality by chartering specific projects to improve processes of critical importance, making improvements using scientific techniques, monitoring the changes, and continually moving on to new projects.

## Nominate Projects

Where does quality improvement make an important difference to a health care organization? The first key step is to select the right topics. Projects should be selected based on evidence that they warrant improvement and will have a visible impact. To nominate projects, it is important to consider existing information that points to quality and cost problems. Consider the following sources:

• *Customers*. Patient complaints and dissatisfaction are critically important. When patients encounter poor quality, most will complain to family, friends, co-workers, and even strangers. Instead of complaining to their doctor or the hospital, many will simply shop around for new caregivers. Any complaint may identify a process needing improvement. But do not rely solely on complaints to learn about customer satisfaction problems. To get a complete and accurate picture, suppliers must seek out information from customers. Actively pursue customer opinions and experiences through survey methods (that address important issues, not just the food and temperature) and focus groups (Nelson and Wasson, 1993).

• *Purchasers*. Health plans and employers are other sources for quality improvement projects. Increasingly they have particular interests and concerns. Many purchasers initiate a dialogue with hospitals and health plans around quality goals. Alternatively, some health plans and hospitals proactively elicit purchaser needs.

• *Suppliers*. As internal suppliers and customers, clinicians can identify care processes with chronic problems. They naturally benchmark in their clinical practice as they discuss cases with colleagues and move from one institutional setting to another. Ask them what worries them about the care their patients receive. Ask them what quality problems they see in processes they work in. These concerns make excellent projects, particularly in the initial stages of building a quality program. Solving problems identified by clinicians helps win their confidence.

• *Reviews and audits*. Use existing data, studies, and reviews from the quality assurance and risk management departments. External data sources may also exist. Often there are old studies that were never acted upon. JCAHO site visits, particularly with the new revised standards, often uncover issues that make for important projects. These types of data can identify deficient processes that need a new approach, something different from that used by previous ineffective improvement efforts.

• *Strategic and annual goals.* Many hospitals and HMOs now set strategic goals related to corporate vision, customer retention, and cost efficiency. Specific projects should be carefully aligned with existing goals. Additionally, annual goals typically translate into specific projects to improve quality of care and outcomes.

## Evaluate Projects

After projects have been nominated, each proposal must be evaluated objectively in terms of potential impact on the following matters:

Improving the health status of the population

Retaining patients, payers, and providers

Attracting new patients, payers, and providers

Reducing deficiencies, waste, and costs of poor quality

Enhancing professional satisfaction

To evaluate possible projects, data on the following four areas are helpful:

1. Complaints and dissatisfaction most likely to drive away existing or new customers
2. The competition's comparative level of quality and cost
3. The most costly and hazardous process deficiencies
4. Deficiencies in internal processes that have the most adverse effect on employees

Specific, objective data are needed on these four areas. Using data is essential for three reasons:

1. Quality improvement is an investment. Be certain to invest in improvements that will lead to meaningful change.

2. Data tell which problems are the most important.

3. Data demonstrate whether the project achieves any improvement.

## Select a Project

Reviewing data on potential projects against specific criteria helps in selecting the most appropriate project. Look at the following seven areas:

1. *How chronic is the problem?* The project should correct a continuing problem, not a recent special episode.

2. *How significant will the results be?* When a project is completed, significant favorable results should be evident. The results should be worth the effort.

3. *Is the project a manageable size?* It should take less than a year for most quality improvement projects to achieve measurable results. Many can be completed in less than six months. If it appears a project will take a long time to complete, it may lack specificity or be more suited for off-line research. It is usually possible to divide such programs into smaller, more narrowly focused projects likely to yield results more quickly.

4. *What is the project's potential impact?* Impact must be measured. Typical measures include the project's potential to retain customers and attract new ones, reduce patient hazard and costs of poor quality, provide return on investment, enhance customer satisfaction, or enhance employee satisfaction.

5. *How urgent is the project to the organization?* A project may be urgent if it addresses quality problems in core services, problems that make the organization highly vulnerable to the competition, or issues that are crucial to key customers.

Problems in these areas are usually critical and should be corrected promptly.

6. *What are the risks?* If there are known or suspected risks, a project is likely to take a long time to complete or have an uncertain outcome. This does not mean the project should be avoided. It simply means the expected payoff should be high. Projects are likely to be risky if they involve new or unproved technology or affect departments that are planning or have recently undergone major organizational changes.

7. *What kinds of resistance might the project create?* Any quality improvement project causes change, and change frequently causes some resistance. The source of resistance may be a difficult manager whose input is important, or an entrenched organizational culture, tradition, or policy. When the choice is among several projects of equal duration, impact, significance, size, urgency, and risk, it is usually best to select the project likely to meet the least resistance.

### When the Organization Is New to Quality Improvement

In organizations relatively new to quality improvement, there are two additional criteria to consider when selecting a project. The first is, the project should be a sure winner. The first projects for an organization new to quality management provide opportunities to learn and adapt the quality improvement process. For this reason, there should be no obstacles in the way of successful outcomes. First projects should still address chronic, significant problems, but not necessarily the *most* significant ones. It is especially important to keep early projects bite-sized and to achieve quick and visible results. Potential impact and urgency are of lesser importance.

Second, the problem must be measurable. All quality improvement projects require measurable problems, but sometimes organizations do not yet have solid data with which to evaluate the potential impact of first projects. Nevertheless, no project should be undertaken if the problem cannot be measured. If no data exist, the project team will need to develop those data during its early work.

## Step 2: Establish a Project

There are three steps to establishing a project once it has been identified: prepare a mission statement, select a project team, and verify the mission.

### Prepare a Mission Statement

The mission statement is the written instruction to the team selected to tackle a quality improvement project. It describes:

The clinical process to be improved

The problem, based on existing data

The objective of the project—what the team is to do about the problem

An effective mission statement clearly identifies the inputs (patient cohort of interest), process of care, and outcomes. It puts the problem in measurable terms, not anecdotes. Finally, the mission statement defines a project that is manageable. It circumscribes the work of the team, distinguishing it from other activities and problems (see Exhibit 6.1).

### Select a Project Team

Successful quality improvement generally requires teams composed of cross-functional groups of people who share the problem and represent various places in the work flow. For example, to ensure optimal outcomes of emergency central line placement, medicine, surgery, anesthesia, nursing, and central supply would be teamed together to diagnose root causes of complications in this process.

Exhibit 6.1. Sample Mission Statement.

State Medicare Peer Review Organization data reveal that Community Health Plan (CHP) has high admission and readmission rates for elderly patients (over seventy-five years old). Specifically, compared to similar populations, CHP members are readmitted for dehydration at significantly higher rates than those on other health plans.

Data suggest that a significant proportion of these admissions are preventable through more aggressive ambulatory management. The most common admitting diagnoses are "failure to thrive" and "dehydration secondary to diuresis." This project team will identify root causes of these admissions and propose changes to ambulatory care that will reduce the frequency of these admissions by one-third in twelve months.

This team approach is important because of the basic structure of health care organizations. Although every hospital and group practice is unique, most are characterized by functional specialization among physicians and vertical lines of authority between nonphysician groups. Typically, individuals do not fully understand one another's roles in patient-care processes. Professionally diverse teams bring very different process knowledge to the improvement team. Patient-care processes flow horizontally through the organization. Individuals from several specialties, departments, and functions interact with the patient. Each step along the way has an impact on the patient. Recall the obstetrical team described earlier, concerned about reducing rates of cesarean section. Figure 6.4 is a process flow diagram demonstrating who should be on the team.

The cross-functional team approach to quality is effective for several reasons. First, team involvement promotes sharing of the problem and minimizes finger pointing. Also, the diversity of team members brings a more complete working knowledge of the process to be improved. Improving a process requires a thorough understanding of how the process works in different areas of the hospital

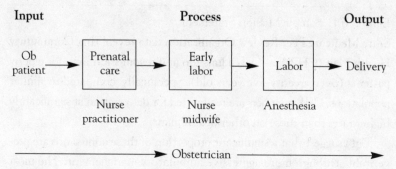

Figure 6.4. Makeup of Cross-Functional C-Section Team.

or health system. Finally, representation from various specialties and departments promotes the acceptance and implementation of change throughout the hospital or clinical unit. Solutions designed with the active participation of affected individuals tend to be technically superior and accepted more readily by those who must implement them.

### Verify the Mission

Once a team meets, its first substantive task is to verify the team mission. This is the final activity for establishing a project, and it requires that the team:

- Verify that the problem exists. The mission statement should include a quantitative description of the problem. If the problem has not been measured, however, the team may need to make measurements before proceeding.

- Identify any aspects of the project that need clarification.

- Verify that the team members represent the appropriate departments and clinical specialties; request that the quality council make adjustments, if needed.

- Clarify the expectations and commitments of team members. Identify the minimum level of involvement for physicians, and define any compensation or release arrangements. Revise the written mission to reflect the precise expectations of the team's work.

## Step 3: Diagnose the Cause

There are five activities to this step:

1. Analyze practice patterns.
2. Identify performance below intention in process of care and outcomes.
3. Formulate hypotheses about causes of outcomes differences and test theories.
4. Test theories with simple, brief data collection or analysis of existing data.
5. Identify root causes such as system barriers and physician practice styles that lead to suboptimal patient outcomes.

Step 3, diagnosing the cause, is analogous to a clinician's use of diagnostic procedures to identify the cause of a patient's symptoms. As with clinical decision making, it is important to establish the cause before prescribing a remedy. If cause is not established, the remedy will probably be ineffective and potentially counterproductive. The difference is that diagnosing process failures and causes of suboptimal outcomes involves looking at practice patterns for cohorts of patients, not just individual cases.

### Tools for Diagnosing Causes of Poor Performance

The diagnostic phase begins with a process flow diagram of the typical care process for the most common cohort of comparable patients. A high-level flow diagram (see Figure 6.5) is a simple tool to summarize the entire care process. A detailed process flow diagram would include several tasks and decision points for prenatal, labor, and delivery management. The process steps most important to identify are those that have been demonstrated to be causally related to outcomes. For example, smoking cessation is a key step in prenatal care that is known to correlate to better pregnancy outcomes. Education of expectant mothers, fathers, and grandparents about the safety of vaginal birth after cesarean deliveries is another process step known to be critical.

Based on the flow diagram, the team generates hypotheses about process deficiencies that may be causing suboptimal performance (see Figure 6.6). Hypotheses address any possible system or attributable cause of practice patterns that can be improved.

### Test Theories

Next, clinical teams must collect data that will enable them to test their hypotheses about causes of variation in practice and outcomes. Testing theories always requires collecting and interpreting data to identify practice patterns that do not contribute to achieving optimal outcomes. Only data that will help identify practice patterns that may be contributing to suboptimal outcomes and that practitioners can control should be collected.

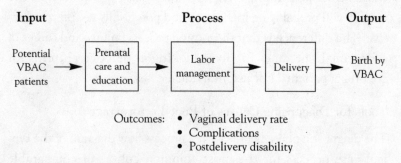

Figure 6.5. High-Level Flow Diagram of C-Section Process.

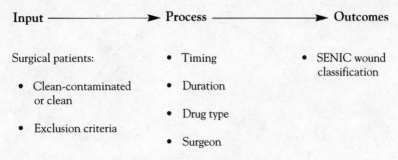

Figure 6.6. Hypotheses About Wound Infections.

It is important to be parsimonious about data collection. Every variable adds cost to the project. It should be clear why each variable is collected and how it will test the team's hypotheses about causes of poor performance. In the C-section example, the team collected data on the process of care and outcomes for repeat C-sections and VBACs performed in the previous year to determine what steps in the process contributed to performing sections rather that VBACs.

## Step 4: Remedy the Cause

Once the root causes are known, clinicians can identify what changes in practice patterns and hospital procedure will result in improved performance. The team should not jump immediately on its first impulse. It is important to consider and evaluate a range of options before selecting one for implementation. This should include a review of the literature on the issue to ensure any existing scientific evidence to support or reject a particular intervention is taken into account. It should also include benchmarking with other organizations that have better cost efficiency and quality performance, to understand their process design.

In some cases, a small pilot is advisable to evaluate the impact of a proposed change (see Figure 6.7). The P-D-C-A cycle applies to projects generally but also to pilots in particular. Teams should

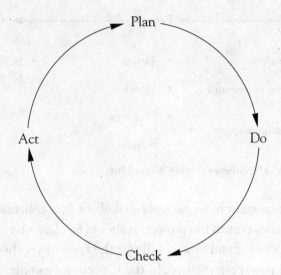

Figure 6.7. Pilot Project.

test and evaluate the impact of their interventions before implementing major changes in care processes. The pilot will help answer these vital questions:

What change in performance is needed?

How will we measure improvement?

Will planned changes lead to improvement (based on scientific knowledge)?

*Hospital Example*

A hospital quality improvement team was assigned the task of reducing the incidence of hospital-acquired urinary tract infections (UTI). The team considered several process changes, including replacing latex foley catheters with silver-lined foley catheters that were being promoted by a medical supply company because they reportedly resulted in fewer infections. Rather than simply adopt the new technology based on a favorable evaluation by the manufacturer, the hospital conducted a simple experiment to prove the efficacy of the new catheter in preventing UTIs. They compared infection rates in uncomplicated patients, giving one cohort latex foleys and another cohort the silver-lined catheters.

The findings of the pilot trial documented that the silver-lined catheters had no impact on the infection rate among women and actually increased the infection rate among men. This pilot trial caused the team to consider other remedies to improve their process of preventing hospital-acquired UTIs.

### Group Practice Example

A capitated group practice wanted to increase the proportion of women over fifty who received mammographic screening exams every two years. The study team hypothesized three alternative remedies and tested them in a comparative pilot. Women in the first group received a personalized reminder letter from their physician. The second received a more formal letter, spelling out the national standards for mammography screening. The third alternative involved administrative assistants in the process by having them personally remind women to get mammograms when they came in for services. The third alternative was far more effective and was selected for implementation.

### Culture Change

An organizational intervention to a care process has its technical aspects, such as new procedures, changes in equipment, or modification of measurements and reports. These technical changes also create changes in the organization's culture. Both aspects of change may cause individuals to resist the proposed changes.

Implementing a remedy for a specific quality problem requires addressing the resistance that the remedy may generate. Implementing quality improvement typically generates resistance to change. It is generally best to minimize the jargon and demonstrate the value of new concepts with actions and examples, not slogans and platitudes.

## Step 5: Hold Gains

After new performance levels are achieved, it is critical to continue to provide feedback to practitioners and to monitor a subset of outcome or process measures routinely. These measures become indicators of performance that are monitored over time to ensure new performance levels are maintained.

A minimum of information is required to accomplish this task, perhaps only one outcome measure or a single process measure. The one caveat is that with summary indicators such as the UTI infection rate or mammography screening rate, the information lacks detail to explain *why* a rate is at a particular level. The level of detail of measures monitoring maintenance is considerably less than that needed when a team is working to diagnose what needs to change.

## Step 6: Replicate Results

Often there will be lessons learned in a project that are highly relevant to other specialties, procedures, and diagnoses. Sometimes the lessons need to be shared with other floors or services within the hospital. Always take the time at the end of a project to identify who can benefit from the knowledge of the team completing its work.

Once this step is completed, it is time to terminate the team. It may play an ongoing periodic role (usually annually) in reviewing the status of outcome measures for the condition or procedure. This is a maintenance function, to interpret maintenance measures and determine if performance has slipped.

## Conclusion

Quality improvement is achieved project by project. Quality improvement projects follow a structured process that relies on simple data collection and many other analytic tools. Results of improvement projects may not be rigorous, publishable new knowledge, but they can lead to improved patient care, patient satisfaction and loyalty, and improved efficiency.

Health care organizations need a systematic approach and infrastructure to support chartering and facilitating teams that achieve measurable results. Initially, when an organization is new to this approach, pilot projects can function independently and be successful. Over time, however, organizations will have dozens of teams, which need to maintain focus and track their impact. This growth can only be managed with a comprehensive plan and strategy. In the advanced stages of TQM implementation, organizations integrate clinical quality and business planning. The next chapter explains how strategic planning can be used by health care organizations.

# 7

Strategic Planning
for Clinical Quality
and Performance

Many health care organizations, like other complex institutions and businesses, have a strategic planning function. Traditionally, the main goal of strategic planning was to evaluate environmental and competitive forces and to craft a high-level plan to steer the entire organization in a successful direction, relative to the competition. Typically, strategic plans were developed by a relatively small number of high-ranking executives within the organization and were not shared with a broad audience of staff. Even today, it is common to have separate planning functions for corporate strategy, finance, and marketing (see Figure 7.1).

Effective planning for clinical quality is a rarity. In health care, more often than not, traditional strategic plans are of little interest or relevance to practitioners.

As the health care reform debate brings the importance of quality and efficiency into focus, many organizations are beginning to develop strategic plans and set goals for quality performance. Some are attempting to integrate strategic, financial, marketing, and quality planning processes (Arvantes, 1993; Veatch, 1993). But how do all these planning activities fit together? What value do they have for patients? For employers and other purchasers? For clinicians?

Learning strategic quality planning requires an entire text of its own. However, this chapter provides an overview of modern

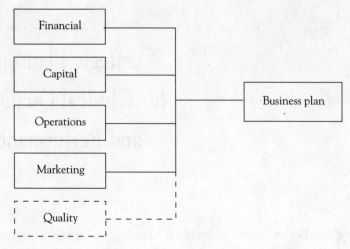

Figure 7.1. Traditional Planning.

strategic planning and identifies how it can be useful to clinicians in managing the quality of patient care and outcomes.

## Strategic Quality Planning

Strategic quality planning (SQP) integrates all aspects of long- and short-range planning into a logical framework. It always derives from a vision statement—an explicit, comprehensive, unique vision of where the organization would like to be in the future. Effective vision statements are customer focused, doable, compelling, and shared throughout the organization. Developing a corporate vision entails a participatory process and requires an investment of time and energy. It can pay off, however, because both the development process and the vision statement itself help to orient the entire organization toward the future and build awareness about necessary change.

Vision statements are little more than wish lists. They do not tell people how to change. Converting a vision of the future into actions people must take is the role of strategic planning. SQP is the process that translates the vision statement into tangible, concrete, measurable goals with explicit time periods. Progress is measured and evaluated against these concrete goals.

### The Essence of Strategic Quality Planning

- Integrates quality, financial, and all other areas

- Focuses on the customer

- Derives from organizational vision

- Involves many in the organization

- Sets explicit goals

- Emphasizes measurable progress

Successful organizations invest in making this process widely participatory rather than strictly top down. This can be one of the most challenging aspects of strategic quality planning for health care organizations, because the notion of a cohesive organization with common vision and goals is new for clinicians. Nonetheless, because they are at the core of the services provided to patients, clinician involvement in strategic planning is critical to successful use of these techniques.

Planning is potentially a painstaking experience, particularly if it is undertaken before an organization has had adequate experience with TQM. To practitioners it can seem to be a bureaucratic exercise that comes out of a corporate office or a lofty distraction from the real business of caring for patients. If modern strategic planning has value to health care organizations, then it must be experienced as meaningful and relevant to practitioners.

The new definition of quality—the presence of desired features and the absence of deficiencies can help to clarify why planning this is so important for clinical quality (see discussion in Chapter Two, particularly Table 2.1). In the past, practicing good medicine meant avoiding or hiding mistakes. Attending a reputable training program, practicing according to the community standards, maintaining current licensure, and avoiding repeated malpractice litigation defined a good doctor. Today, there are many more dimensions of the definition of quality and performance. Avoiding being an outlier on objective performance measures is quality at a minimum. Competing on quality requires much more.

*Freedom from deficiency* means avoiding mistakes, but increasingly it also means practice consistent with explicit clinical guidelines and continuous improvements that are invisible to patients. In the future there will be more and more objective performance measures to evaluate practice patterns and outcomes relative to peer organizations. *Features* refers to care designed to meet the complex and perhaps conflicting needs of multiple patient and payer groups. It means using sophisticated communication techniques to involve patients in decision making. It also means caring for patients and preventing health problems in ways the public cannot even imagine. It even means finding ways to demonstratively change the health status of communities.

This definition of quality, which adds the dimension of cost efficiency to the equation, reflects a much more comprehensive view of health systems. It presumes an epidemiologic approach and systems thinking about communities and customers. It is within this context that clinicians need to work with others in health organizations to plan for their future role within their communities.

## When and How to Plan

Comprehensive, participatory strategic quality planning can be an important element in an overall TQM program for health care organizations. The key is to engage in integrated strategic quality planning when it is right for an individual organization.

After the broad base of leadership has come to understand the basic quality management approach and comprehends the value of an overall strategy, a planning process involving clinicians as well as other professionals and employees may be useful. If the department chairs need evidence that TQM has something to offer them and demand documentation of its value, leave strategic and financial planning processes as they currently exist until the base of support for TQM has grown. For a strategic planning effort to be effective, participants must have sufficient experience conducting quality projects to understand the value of systematic planning. It takes experience with several projects before clinicians and other staff recognize the need for a logical and cohesive plan that frames all the projects and connects them to the strategic goals and the vision.

### Policies Affecting Quality

One important issue to consider when undertaking strategic quality planning is policies within an organization and the degree to which they support the new planning process. A comprehensive planning process may be desirable, but if staff are working under managed-care contracts and compensation policies that create conflicts or resistance to TQM, these policies may need to be modified before a planning process is undertaken.

### Overview of the Planning Process

The general approach to planning entails several phases and components (see Figure 7.2). First, there is the decision to plan, described above. This will be unique for every organization. Timing is critical, particularly as it relates to involving clinicians. Also, planning needs to be viewed as an iterative process; strategic planning continuously improves, like all processes in TQM organizations. Identifying incremental changes that will be embraced by a broad base within the organization should dictate the pace and style of change in the planning process.

Second, there needs to be careful assessment of the organization's current level of performance relative to its long-term vision.

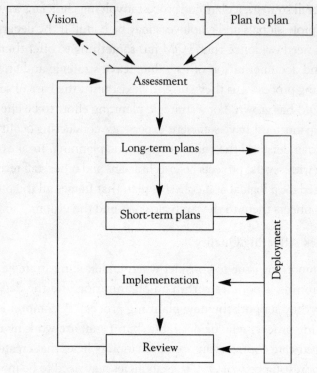

Figure 7.2.  General Planning Model.

This is done with existing information. Invariably this assessment unleashes criticisms about existing performance information on quality of care and services. It is important to separate the discussion of improving performance information and information systems from planning strategic goals. Most organizations cannot afford to postpone strategic quality planning until they have a perfect information system. However, many organizations need to address their information capabilities as part of their long- and short-term plans.

The assessment leads to the sequential derivation of long-term and short-term plans. Both of these must be deployed, meaning that they must be assigned to specific individuals and groups along with necessary resources for implementation. Finally, plans must be reviewed at regular intervals to evaluate progress.

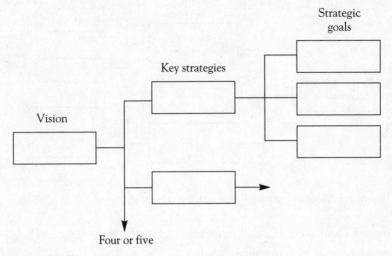

Figure 7.3. Tree Diagram for Long-Term Planning.

The basic tool for strategic planning is the tree diagram, like the one in Figure 7.3. It provides a framework for identifying and documenting the means required to achieve a specific objective.

Key strategies and goals represent specific objectives that, when implemented, will provide evidence that the organization has achieved its vision. Implementation of a strategic plan requires breaking down strategic goals (objectives) into the activities (means) required to achieve those goals (see Figure 7.4). These activities are the projects that enable organizations to realize key strategies and, ultimately, their vision. By breaking the goals and subgoals into small components, the work can be assigned to individuals and teams for completion.

Tree diagrams can be used at the summary level (as in Figure 7.3) as well as the detail level (Figure 7.5). The value of a tree diagram is that it demonstrates logical connections between the vision, strategies, goals, and projects. The diagram displays how each detailed project or activity rolls up into broad goals that relate directly to the vision. Because the vision represents a dramatic departure from the status quo and therefore requires major change to achieve, it is crucial to persuade everyone that the sum of all

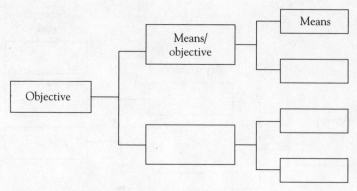

Figure 7.4.  Means Sum to Achieve Objectives.

projects and activities will in fact be successful. Tree diagrams help communicate this message.

### Case Example: An HMO Strategic Plan

Consider a health plan serving 100,000 members in a suburban area in the Southwest. It vision includes becoming dominant in the region, a fully capitated HMO with an integrated delivery system led by a physician-hospital organization. While it will continue to serve patients of all ages, the HMO is committed to becoming the area's market leader in senior care. Part of the vision seeks demonstrably to improve the health of its membership. Key strategies include an initiative targeted at the large Medicare population under risk contract with the Health Care Financing Administration. One strategic goal might be measurably to improve the functional status of members over age seventy-five. One subgoal of this strategy could be implementing a case management and patient empowerment program for patients with chronic illnesses. Annual goals might specifically address reducing admissions for drug complications, increasing patients' satisfaction with their participation in treatment decisions, and decreasing inappropriate use of invasive cardiac procedures.

Another strategic goal might be to improve pregnancy outcomes among plan members. A subgoal that could lead to this objective

Objective – Means

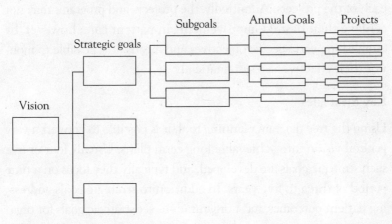

Figure 7.5.  Deploying the Vision.

would be to reduce the occurrence of low-birth-weight babies by 10 percent. This subgoal can be achieved through two means: reducing the incidence of preterm labor by 50 percent and lowering the rate of smoking among pregnant women by 25 percent.

A third example of a subgoal might be to reduce the functional disability, severity of acute exacerbations, and total cost of managing asthma. This subgoal will result from the following projects:

Increasing the knowledge level of patients with asthma by 25 percent

Increasing the use of inhaled steroids by 50 percent

Increasing the use of home nebulizers by 33 percent

Designing, implementing, and monitoring a protocol and care process of office emergency care

It should be possible to summarize a strategic plan into high-level goals and subgoals and to drill down into the details of individual projects and activities. Annual goals can be translated into detailed project statements, and teams can be chartered to achieve measurable results. Individuals can be assigned accountability for each of the projects. Admittedly, the projects and programs may not achieve their desired improvements in patient care; however, by establishing very specific objectives and means, it is possible to monitor their effectiveness systematically.

## Key Strategies

Using the tree diagram planning tool, it is possible to convert a very general vision into achievable long-term plans. Usually four or five such strategic goals are developed, and typically they focus on a time period of three to five years. In addition to strategic goals addressing patient outcomes, most organizations set strategic goals for organizational structure and governance (for-profit or not-for-profit), desired configuration (staff-model HMO, mixed-model HMO, types of networks and institutional relationships), and preferred customer base (target purchasers and members).

## Setting Short-Term Goals

After long-term strategic initiatives have been identified, short-term quality goals should be set. The time frame for achieving these goals is usually one year. Setting annual goals is the second step in converting a vision into operational plans (see Figure 7.5). These quantitative goals guide the organization's budget allocations, team assignments, and should result in achievement of each key long-term strategy.

Setting annual quality goals requires specific information on the organization's performance relative to comparable organizations and customer priorities and requirements. Consider a community hospital that provides cardiac surgery for a significant number of people. This "product line" constitutes 25 percent of the hospital's revenues under fee-for-service, and increasingly local payers are interested in bundled fees based on competitive bids. Therefore improving performance in this clinical area is a strategic initiative.

Suppose the length of stay was on average 4.3 days longer than hospitals elsewhere and the risk-adjusted mortality was slightly higher than the national average. To achieve parity with peers in other markets in all cardiac surgery services, the hospital might set annual goals like these:

- Reduce average length of stay for cardiac surgery care by 25 percent.

- Reduce complication rates for cardiac surgery patients to parity with market leaders.

- Increase cardiac surgery patient satisfaction by 10 percent per year.

### Subject Matter of Strategic Quality Goals

Selecting the right goals to focus on is an issue for serious consideration. Five general topics are important to consider.

#### Customer Satisfaction

In many market areas, there are purchasers who are prepared to identify their priorities and concerns. They may have analyzed their health care expenditures and want to provide input on hospital or managed-care organization's goals. For example, many purchasers are particularly interested in the cost and quality of hospital care. Others are more concerned with mental health episodes of illness or work-related injuries. Some purchasers are actually making their own assessments about the quality and efficiency of various providers and managed-care organizations.

Often businesses are not organized into one voice and therefore it is more difficult to assess their needs. Identifying purchasers' concerns and addressing them in long-term and short-term goals is critically important.

In some regions of the country, public advocate organizations such as the American Association of Retired Persons represent the interests of individual patients and members. In general, the public as consumer and patient has been less directly involved than employers in the debate on health care quality measurement and public disclosure of performance information at the local level. Some peer review organizations, charged with representing the interests of the elderly in assessing the quality delivered under the Medicare program, actively solicit the needs and concerns of the patients.

Not surprisingly, consumers often take quality for granted when it comes to health care. Because it is a negative purchase, meaning it is something to be avoided, most advocacy groups are formed around a particular condition such as muscular dystrophy, arthritis, or cancer. Eliciting the needs and interests of patient groups in order to use this information in strategic planning may warrant targeted efforts by diagnosis group. In general, this type of customer needs assessment work is new to clinicians.

### Outcomes Quality

This type of goal relates to level of deficiencies and quality of performance. Outcomes quality goals may address processes that are highly visible and understandable for patients or they may refer to technical quality that is assumed by patients or beyond their comprehension. This type of goal may address performance on publicly reported measures or major performance features with direct visibility to patients and payers, such as service behavior of professionals and employees, waiting times, accuracy of patient information, patient confidentiality, and safety.

Any aspect of service or clinical quality that directly affects patients and their judgments about the organization is a prime candidate. Health status and clinical outcomes performance are somewhat more removed but also reflect on the overall performance of the organization.

### Cost of Poor Quality (COPQ)

Because of the tremendous public concern about health care costs as well as widespread perception and evidence of waste in the health care system, focusing toward reducing unnecessary or undesirable utilization and cost to purchasers is an excellent choice for strategic goals. For example, many managed-care organizations expend administrative resources micromanaging providers. This activity is typically redundant to managerial activities internal to the provider organizations. Reducing this type of administrative cost by partnerships focused on improving efficiency would be an excellent choice for a strategic initiative. For a hospital, identifying areas where fixed payer margins or capitation are driving down revenues is an important topic for strategic and annual goals.

Juran Institute consultants perform COPQ analyses to determine where an organization is losing money or market share and creating quality hazards for patients. In nearly every organization studied to date, the opportunities to improve care and enhance efficiency appear for clinical cohorts where there is high variation in practice patterns. For these clinical conditions, the rewards for meeting strategic goals will be high.

### Competitive Performance

Competitive quality performance should be a part of the strategic quality plan. This requires knowing the performance level and service features of competitors. Goals of this type explicitly target improving performance relative to competitor organizations on some important dimension of service or quality.

### Performance of Administrative Processes

Administrative functions that support the quality and efficiency of health care are important topics for strategic initiatives. There is tremendous public concern over the percentage of the health care budget going to administrative overhead rather than services. Demonstrating high performance in this area is extremely timely for health care organizations. Information systems are particularly important administrative functions within health care that are significantly underdeveloped relative to current needs.

### Deployment of Goals

The deployment of goals entails a management process to track progress against the plan. This requires detailed administrative support to ensure that each project achieves its intended results. Each project leader needs a work plan, which will vary by project type. Planning projects (see Chapter Five) may require more time and support. Measurement and quality control activities may be required on an ongoing basis (see Chapter Four). Likewise, quality improvement project leaders need to lay out a work plan that investigates root causes and defines ways to measurably improve care and outcomes (see Chapter Six).

## Review Process

A formal, efficient review process will increase the probability of reaching your organization's goals. The key is to identify measures of progress that can be monitored over time. Frequent measurement of progress displayed in graphic form helps to identify the gaps in need of attention. When the improvement goal is clear and well accepted, such as increasing the proportion of children immunized according to the American Academy of Pediatrics, monitoring progress against stated goals will increase the likelihood of success. A worksheet like that displayed in Exhibit 7.1 is a valuable tool.

Exhibit 7.1. Strategic Goal Worksheet.

Strategic Goal: _____

Strategy Leader: _____

| | | Supporting Projects | | | | |
|---|---|---|---|---|---|---|
| Subgoals | Annual goals | Project | Leader | Baseline measurement | Target | Completion date |
| | | | | | | |
| | | | | | | |
| | | | | | | |
| | | | | | | |
| | | | | | | |
| | | | | | | |
| | | | | | | |
| | | | | | | |
| | | | | | | |

## Barriers to Clinician Involvement

There are a number of cultural and professional barriers to strategic planning for clinicians. Most important, clinical training fosters the belief that the clinician's *only* role is to care for individual patients when they are ill. This leads to a reactive role, which makes proactive thinking and planning for health of patient populations difficult. In addition, knowledge of systems, epidemiology, and management of organizations are considered "electives" for clinicians. They are not treated as subjects all practitioners should understand or master.

Later in the process of strategic planning, clinicians within and between specialties need to identify the core processes affecting their patients. The core clinical processes may be diagnosis specific (such as the prevention or care of asthma, coronary artery disease, or cancer) or they may be generic or independent of diagnoses (such as hemodynamic stability management, anesthesia management, patient education). It is extremely helpful to the organization as a whole for clinicians within and between specialties to identify their core processes. Strategic and annual goals will lay the groundwork for selecting core processes for which resources are to be invested for quality measurement, planning, and improvement.

Some organizations have found it useful to engage clinicians in a process of identifying their core processes that have greatest impact on their community before undertaking strategic planning. This may prove useful early on in the implementation of TQM to help clinicians focus on processes and populations of patients.

For example, consider an IPA HMO whose vision is to become the most desirable source of primary care for young families in its region. Pediatricians in an affiliated group practice need to identify their core processes that must improve dramatically as part of the overall strategic initiative. They might develop a list like this:

Providing telephone advice

Diagnosis and treatment of otitis media

Diagnosis and treatment of asthma

Well-child care

Accident prevention

Every clinical service of a group practice or hospital should undertake the same step of identifying its most important processes. Some critical processes will cross specialties, such as the management of menopause, which involves internal medicine, gynecology, and endocrinology. Identifying core processes can be done before or during strategic planning for clinical quality.

## Conclusion

For organizations at an advanced stage of quality management, strategic planning provides a framework to accelerate and focus their progress. Strategic planning requires a readiness for systems thinking on the part of clinicians. It calls for identifying the core processes of clinical care for the organization as a whole, within and between specialties. SQP tools include various tree diagrams and matrices to display the relationship between the vision, strategic goals, annual goals, and projects, down to the level of frequent measurements of progress.

Typically, organizations do not attempt strategic planning until the later stages of TQM implementation. The next chapter describes the stages of implementation and the components that must be addressed at each stage of development.

# 8

. . . . . . . . . . . . . . . . . . . . . . . . . .

# Implementing
# Quality Management
# in Clinical Settings

As clinicians prepare to assume management roles in clinical delivery systems such as physician hospital organizations, group practices, and managed-care organizations, they often wonder, "How can I be successful?" This chapter delineates the five phases of implementation and practical steps needed during each phase. This implementation plan is designed to serve as a roadmap for leaders as they begin to direct their clinical quality programs.

*Five Implementation Phases*

. . . . . . . . . . . . . . . . . . . . . . . . . . . . . .

1. Decide.

2. Prepare.

3. Start.

4. Expand.

5. Integrate.

*Deciding* to implement total quality management requires an assessment of the drivers for change (see Chapter One) and an understanding of how this approach differs from other management approaches, including quality assurance. *Preparing* to implement a comprehensive strategy to manage cost and quality requires clinicians

This chapter was written by Robert B. Halder, M.D.

to lay out an implementation plan, select clinician leaders for training in special skills, and establish some initial clinical cost and quality goals. *Starting* implementation involves establishing pilot care-improvement teams and creating an infrastructure to support clinical measurement and improvement activities. During the *expansion* phase, organizations assess pilot project results and identify lessons learned. Successes are communicated widely to clinical staff and more clinicians become involved in new projects. Finally, during the *integration* phase, clinicians participate with administrators and other managers to integrate clinical and nonclinical projects into an organizationwide strategic plan.

Many hospitals and health maintenance organizations have successfully implemented quality management programs in administration and service. Far fewer have succeeded at implementation in clinical care. In the long run, organizations that apply continuous improvement throughout their organizations will achieve stronger community reputations and greater market share.

## Phase 1: Decide on a Quality Management Approach

Purchaser and patient awareness of their powerful role as customers, market competition, and cost pressures drive many health care organizations to evaluate their approach to managing quality.

### Partial Approaches

Seeing no other options, many clinicians respond to the driving forces for change (see Chapter One) by using the traditional quality assurance model. Its prime customers are regulators. The approach is typically reactive. The focus is on the individual physician or case rather than on cohorts of patients. It focuses on idealized processes. The methodology is based on inspection and feedback and its use of statistics is limited. While the quality assurance model has been successful in meeting yesterday's requirements, it requires expansion to meet the challenges facing clinicians today.

Another partial approach has been the formation of clinician-led task forces designed to meet with regulators and buyers for the purpose of buying time and negotiating for the minimum amount of intrusion on the status quo. Sophisticated customers soon see right through this strategy. Some clinicians and their administrators are promising to measure and reduce costs but lack the knowledge and commitment to do so.

Many clinicians are negotiating for capitated rates—which they know cannot be profitable—hoping that cost shifting will save them. Typically this fails. Yesterday's margin and yesterday's options are gone.

Some clinicians close their private practices and hire on with health maintenance organizations and preferred provider organizations, hoping that the challenges will go away.

These partial approaches will not work because they do not produce the basic clinical cost, patient satisfaction, and functional outcomes that patients and buyers want and clinicians need in order to stay competitive.

## TQM as a Solution

Many health care organizations respond to the driving forces for change by implementing continuous improvement or TQM. TQM is different from traditional quality assurance (see Table 8.1). It systematically addresses the needs of internal and external customers. It offers proactive strategies and techniques that focus on process capability rather than individual clinician deficiencies. It requires pervasive use of epidemiology, statistics, and population-level process and outcomes measurement.

### Tasks for Leaders

During the decide phase, clinical leaders conduct a self-assessment of the current quality performance of their organizations. This should be done in collaboration with administrative leadership. Self-assessment should address questions such as these:

Table 8.1. Quality Assurance and TQM Compared.

|  | Quality Assurance | TQM |
|---|---|---|
| Customers | Regulators | Internal/external |
| Motivation | Reactive | Proactive |
| Performance | Individual | Process |
| Process approach | Idealized | Actual |
| Method | Inspection/Feedback | Data-driven/<br>Process improvement |
| Use of statistics | Limited | Pervasive |

What are the results of recent internal and external quality reviews?

How is our competition performing?

What are the measurable results in process and outcomes of care?

How does the medical staff feel about practicing here?

Are we meeting our customers' expectations in quality and cost?

What is our accreditation status?

Formal self-assessment tools exist (see SunHealth Alliance, 1994). Answering these questions thoroughly using a formal process will provide leadership with an analysis of the organization's current strengths and weaknesses.

Next, clinical leaders should learn about alternative management approaches. Attending conferences on continuous improvement and quality management such as those sponsored by the Joint Commission on Accreditation of Healthcare Organizations (JCAHO) or the Institute for Healthcare Improvement (IHI), reading relevant professional publications (*Quality Connection, Journal on Quality Improvement, Joint Commission Perspectives, Strategies for Healthcare Excellence, The Quality Letter for Healthcare Leaders,* and *Managed Care Medicine*), and talking with peers inside and outside the organization can go a long way in pointing out the best approach to meet the challenges. Armed with this information, clinical leaders must decide which approach to follow and commit to providing the time and resources needed for success.

*Tasks for Clinical Leaders During the Decision Phase*

- Consider organization's current performance in clinical quality.

- Become knowledgeable in the options.

- Select approach to implement.

- Commit the time and resources needed for implementation.

In the climate of shrinking resources and precious little time to commit to new strategies, the decision to implement a comprehensive quality management program is not to be taken lightly. The investment of time and resources is substantial. The benefits must be targeted and essential to the organization's future, and the prospective gains must be communicated as the rationale for the undertaking. The time and resources can often come from other activities that are yielding little value.

## Phase 2: Prepare for Implementation

The overall flow of activity in Phase 2 can be summarized as follows:

- Educate clinic leaders and managers.

- Form quality council, appoint quality executive and staff, and provide training in quality processes to selected leaders.

- Develop explanation of need, vision statement, and quality goals.

- Prepare long-range and annual goals.

- Select pilot projects and teams.

- Communicate actions to clinicians and staff.

## Education

The initial step during the preparation phase is for top management—both clinical and administrative—to become grounded in the fundamentals of TQM. It is important that this management team understand both the clinical and administrative relevance and application of TQM. An off-site interactive educational opportunity, with minimum interruption by pagers and telephones, affords the best chance for success.

## Steering Group

Following this, a top-level team should assume responsibility for directing the TQM activities of the organization. Membership on this steering group, sometimes called the quality council, should include the chief executive officer, the chief operating officer, the senior vice presidents (including the senior nurse), the chief medical officer or director, the president and president-elect of the medical staff, and the quality executive officer. Although organizations may customize the steering group membership to meet their specific structure and needs, the point here is that the most senior administration and clinical leadership must participate to ensure success.

If none exists, a quality executive officer position should be created. Selecting an individual who is knowledgeable in TQM and who can report directly to the chair of the steering group is critical to the success of TQM. Depending on the size of the organization, this officer may require some support staff. Many organizations, as they integrate quality assurance with TQM, find that the former quality assurance director and staff fit well into the roles of TQM executive and staff. Again, these and other selected managers should participate in the early phases of training for quality.

## Vision and Goals

Once formed, the steering group must develop the organization's initial quality goals and quality vision. These represent the desired future state of the organization and should reflect an understanding of what it will take to survive in today's health care market. For example, a vision might be "to be reorganized as the provider of choice in our regional marketplace." The initial goals to support this vision might be these:

1. Analyze customers' needs through proactive dialogue.
2. Develop an organizational infrastructure to begin to address unmet customer needs.
3. Improve customer satisfaction by 10 percent in the next fiscal year.

Being initial goals and vision, these will require refinement and increasing detail and accountability over time. The vision and goals should be woven into the long-range plan for the organization. This plan should place timelines for issues such as training in improvement, planning, and benchmarking as well as establish the details for the first year's rollout. An example of a first-year plan is seen in Table 8.2.

## Pilot Projects and Teams

The highlight of the preparation phase is the selection of pilot improvement projects and teams. These teams, the lessons they learn, and the results they demonstrate will establish TQM as the strategy of choice to meet the challenges facing health care organizations. It is important, therefore, to select these teams wisely.

In the past, the tendency has been to select primarily administrative projects for these pilots. This falls short of the mark. These pilots should include some highly visible care improvement projects. For instance, if the steering group selects four teams, two might target improvements in clinical quality and efficiency, such

Table 8.2. One-Year Roadmap.

| 1 | 2 | 3 | 4 | 5 | 6 | 7 | 8 | 9 | 10 | 11 | 12 |
|---|---|---|---|---|---|---|---|---|----|----|----|
| Executive dialog and assessment | Educate top management | Establish Quality Council | Set quality visions and goals | | Establish project nomination methods | | On-going selection of projects | Establish measures for organization performance | Plan communication strategy | | Communicate results |
| | | | | Train pilot team facilitators | | | Select and train next facilitators | | | | Review results |
| | | | Solicit nominations for pilot teams | Select pilot teams | Train pilot team members | | | | | | |
| | | | | | Train middle managers; clinician leaders | | | | | | |
| | | | | | Introduce TQM to medical staff | | | | | | |
| | | | Review recent customer surveys | Assess the internal culture | | Formally assess market standing | | Begin to look at costs of poor quality | | Begin integration of TQM with JCAHO/NCQA requirements | |

as reducing C-section rates and increasing appropriate use of emergency room services.

Pilot projects can be selected as a result of a nomination process in which clinical leadership plays a key role. The projects should represent clearly recognized chronic quality problems that are measurable and are fixable. Selected pilot projects should relate to top diagnoses and conditions and meet at least the following criteria:

The problems are highly visible and significant.

They are related to customer requirements.

There is a high likelihood for measurable impact in six months.

Success is likely.

The steering group charters pilot teams. Eight to ten people across departments are asked to spend up to three to four hours per week for six to nine months solving a well-defined and specific problem. This is a significant commitment of time and resources, especially for clinicians. Many organizations involve physicians one or two hours every other week as consultants to teams.

The projects should be well developed with supporting data, trained facilitators, and an explicit, quantitative mission statement. A mission statement should include very specific data, goals, interventions, and expectations so that the team understands its purpose and intended results (see also Chapter Six). For example, a project for a hospital might have this mission statement: "Reduce average length of stay for normal vaginal deliveries by 50 percent and increase overall patient satisfaction with obstetrics through innovative educational and home health services." An HMO mission statement might read: "Reduce the admission rate for children with asthma by 25 percent through analyzing practice patterns, identifying best office practices and home care practices, and educating providers and families about prevention strategies."

Selecting members for these pilot teams requires careful planning. The steering group should, at a minimum, name the leaders
and facilitators of the pilot teams. The chemistry between these
individuals is important. Clinical improvement teams should have
clinician team leaders who have a passionate desire to fix the
chronic quality problem at hand. Also, team leaders should be
objective in problem analysis and skillful in group dynamics and
teamwork.

An effective clinical pilot team facilitator may be a clinician but
must be someone with several days' training and experience with
problem analysis, experimental design, and team-building skills.
Taking the time during steering group meetings to select the right
project, the right team leader, and the right facilitator optimizes the
chances for success of pilot teams.

Most steering groups delegate the selection of pilot team members to the appropriate vice president and the medical director or
their subordinates. The key issue here is to select those individuals
who, based upon the steering group's understanding of the process
to be improved, bring the right knowledge base and interpersonal
skills to the project.

## Communication

Activities of the preparation phase should be fully communicated
to upper management, both clinical and administrative. The goal
here is to keep leadership informed and to create an anticipation
that results are coming and that when they arrive, they will be
communicated to the entire organization. At this point it is not
too early to provide the general medical staff with a brief overview
on clinical improvement and TQM and to inform them about the
pilot improvement teams. This introduction may help to identify
some early clinical champions who will serve on future project
teams and possibly enroll in future clinical quality and TQM
training.

*Tasks for Clinical Leaders During the Preparation Phase*

- Become trained in management approach.

- Serve on steering group.

- Establish quality officer.

- Set initial goals and vision.

- Select pilot project or projects.

- Charter pilot project teams.

- Charter assessment and planning task forces.

- Develop first-year plan in detail.

Note that these tasks are nondelegable. Relegating these duties to nonclinicians sends the wrong message to the medical staff and to other clinicians as well. However, early involvement by clinicians in this preparation phase demonstrates that they are going to be the change agents, and facilitates the expanded involvement of clinicians that will be necessary during the next phase.

## Phase 3: Starting the Implementation

During the "start" phase, organizations conduct their pilot projects and build basic infrastructure to support the continuous quality activities.

### Conduct Pilot Projects

Doing the work of the pilot project itself has three phases:

1. Train facilitators, team leaders, and team members.
2. Complete the project.
3. Develop and share the lessons learned.

First, the facilitators, team leaders, and team members selected to conduct the pilot projects require special training. Facilitators must develop skills to enable them to support teams to achieve successful results. Basic tools of quality must be learned, including cause-and-effect analysis, data collection and analysis, and problem solving.

Training should also include understanding team dynamics and practicing the art of facilitating a heterogeneous group toward the accomplishment of a common goal. Facilitators must advise the team leader and team members as to the appropriate tools to use at varying stages of the problem-solving process. The quality officer should have the experience to coach facilitators through the first projects.

The team leaders and team members will require, at a minimum, some basic understanding of team dynamics and basic clinical measurement and quality improvement tools. It helps to provide these pilot teams with one or two days of this training up front, followed by "just-in-time" training on new tools and techniques during team meetings over time. Introducing teams to a mock project and walking the team through a case study illustrate the measurement, analysis, and improvement steps experienced by teams during the problem-solving process. Upon completing this training they usually overcome some of the uncertainty inherent in applying new techniques in a setting with new people. Ongoing training provides reinforcement and expansion of skills.

Next, the team gets to work on the pilot project. For the next six to nine months these trained, facilitated teams work to achieve the goals of their project mission statement. They will come to the steering group with questions and provide interim progress reports. Typically teams experience periods of frustration as they learn complex new skills and new ways to solve problems. Pilot team facilitators will probably develop their own support group to help each other through difficult team issues. Lack of team focus or poor attendance will have to be addressed by team leaders. Teams may have to be reconstituted because of unforeseen logistic or interpersonal difficulties.

If properly selected and supported, most pilot teams will achieve measurable results. All teams will gain invaluable experience that cannot be learned from textbooks and should be shared with others.

## Build Basic Infrastructure

While pilot teams are conducting their projects, the steering group builds a basic infrastructure to support the ongoing quality activities of the organization.

### Assess Quality Status

The first task is to assess the current quality status, which involves examining market share, customer satisfaction, the organization's culture, and existing quality systems.

Clinical leaders should participate in an analysis of the organization's current market standing (see also Chapter Seven). Questions to ask include these:

> How do our occupancy rates, our C-section rates, our average lengths of stay, and our costs per case for certain diagnostic-related groups compare to those of the other hospitals or managed-care organizations in town?

> What is our cost per episode of outpatient care of adult asthma? How does it compare?

> Can we measure cost and quality of care? Can our competitors?

> Can we document improvement over time?

Clinicians should engage in ongoing, proactive dialogue with purchasers to stay informed of their assessments and their specific concerns about particular patient groups or diagnosis.

An important area affecting market share is the cost of poor quality (COPQ). Clinical leaders should work closely with administration, especially the information departments and the quality department staff, to determine high-risk, high-volume, high-resource utilization and high internal variation diagnoses and procedures. A good practice pattern tracking capability, patient-based cost accounting system, and case mix or severity-adjustment system will ensure that data analyses are valid and relevant. Chapter Four discusses some of the measurement and analysis challenges.

Choosing what to monitor at the steering group level is an important element of the start phase. This group should monitor those areas key to the success of the organization. Teams measure these key indicators of organizational performance as defined by payers, regulators, and patients and report results to the steering group on an ongoing basis.

Irrespective of the setting—hospital, HMO, IPA, PPO, or group practice—these clinical measures should reflect those areas key to the success of the organization, and clinical leaders should lead the development of these measures. They may, in addition, be cascaded into the organization and drive department-level measures.

Another aspect in this stage is understanding the internal culture of an organization. This is particularly important when leadership is considering major changes in management approach. The decision to implement a quality management program represents such a major change for most organizations. A thorough understanding of the internal culture can help to facilitate the process.

The goal here is to understand the enablers for change as well as the barriers. Cultural assessment can be conducted by an external consultant with specific expertise. Alternatively, it can be performed by professionals internal to the organization. It usually entails a series of interviews to elicit insights from the spectrum of staff into how this particular organization works, how people communicate, how they solve problems, how they value each other, and what they fear most about change. Understanding the culture will go a long way in overcoming resistance to cultural change.

During the start phase it is also important to assess the current quality system: the infrastructure already in place that is designed to determine what should be measured, how the data is to be collected, and what use will be made of that data once collected. The steering group, with its nondelegable roles, is the key component of this system. Assessment of the role of utilization management, risk management, and the quality assurance activities will reveal ways in which one can start to integrate and coordinate these activities with the new quality management activities.

Additionally, clinical leadership will want to ensure that information management and education and training activities are used to support quality management implementation. The key challenge is to institute changes that eliminate or reduce activities that do not add value to the overall quality program without disrespecting individual contributors. Clinical leaders working in collaboration with these knowledgeable professionals can optimize the output of current activities and reduce activity where it is wasteful or counterproductive.

## Revise Management Systems

The next major element of work in the start phase is reviewing whether any changes in management systems are needed, particularly changes in human resources, management information, and suppliers. Clinical leaders will want to influence any revision of management systems.

During this phase, the human resource department typically redesigns job descriptions to bring expectations into line with the new skill requirements of quality management. This lays the groundwork to recruit and train for the skills necessary to work effectively on cross-functional teams. Clinical leaders will want to participate in these decisions. Restructuring care delivery into a patient-focused care paradigm should be factored in to job expectations as well.

This new array of cross-functional, data-driven activities must be supported by the organization's management information department. Information services must design a system to understand and meet the needs of its clinical customers. This means that clinical leaders work with data managers to devise access, storage, extraction, and analysis capabilities. Data bases need to accommodate software for case mix and risk adjustment. As customers, clinicians must clearly articulate what they need and provide constructive feedback as to how well these needs are being met.

Clinicians with expertise in computer applications, data analysis, and epidemiology can make a major contribution advising in this area. They can also serve as consultants to fellow clinicians, especially clinical leaders, who may not be as familiar with computers, data, and epidemiologic principles. This collaboration can help to overcome resistance to becoming a data-driven organization. Appropriately, clinicians want reassurance from trustworthy peers about the validity, relevance, and confidence levels of data used for any quality monitoring or performance assessments.

Review of supplier relationships is another important area for possible revision. Many suppliers of medical goods and services such as pharmaceutical companies and medical equipment companies have successfully implemented TQM in their own organizations. They are often willing to provide their people to serve as team members or ad hoc consultants to quality improvement teams. For example, a clinical improvement team attempting to decrease the complication rates of central venous catheterization might use catheter suppliers as ad hoc contributors in order to expand the team's understanding of the role the catheters might play in the process under study. Suppliers can often bring a knowledge of clinical processes critical to the redesign of a defective process. This is another area in which leaders can facilitate new levels of cooperation between the organization and those traditionally maintained at a distance.

Another key area of supplier system review and revision is the concept of preferred suppliers. Instead of dealing with literally hundreds of different vendors, why not select a vital few who will give best prices, best service, and best cooperation? Many industries have found this practice extremely cost effective. In addition, it optimizes the chances that what we get is exactly what we ordered.

A final note on supplier relationships: clinicians should period-ically review orders to ensure that the number and features of med-ical devices are kept at an absolute minimum. Clinicians can achieve major cost savings by reducing unnecessary redundancies in supplies. The start phase is a perfect time for clinical leaders to stimulate a review of ordering practices, whether for pharmaceu-ticals or medical equipment and devices.

Another major customer-supplier relationship exists between hos-pitals and managed-care organizations. There are vast opportunities to reduce wasteful administrative costs through performance-based partnerships that strive to eliminate wasteful micromanagement of clinical decision making. There are also fruitful partnerships focused on building data infrastructure for quality management.

### Create Ongoing Processes

Once the first two tasks have been completed—assessing current status of quality and revising management systems—the next crit-ical aspect of the start phase is to create a process by which projects are nominated, selected, assigned, and reviewed on an ongoing basis (see Chapter Six).

Several sources of project candidates have already been men-tioned. Solicitation of projects from all employees via a process improvement opportunity form may also be effective. These forms can be conveniently located throughout the organization, includ-ing the doctors' and nurses' lounges, and submitted to the quality officer. These forms should ask:

What do you see as a chronic quality or waste problem?

Do data exist to support that this is a chronic quality or waste problem?

Would you be willing to serve on a team to solve this problem?

Who else would you suggest might serve on such a team?

How can we contact you?

These solicitations, along with ideas from other sources, can then be collated by the quality staff and presented to the steering group for consideration. Leadership should look at the suggested project and supporting data and then prioritize and select projects (see Chapter Six).

Once projects have been selected, the steering group assigns teams, leaders, and facilitators, writes mission statements, and reviews progress on an ongoing basis. This process becomes a major agenda item for steering group meetings.

## Communicate Results

The completion of the start phase is the time to communicate to the organization the results of pilot projects, lessons learned, updated rollout plans, and new infrastructure built to support the program. This process is critically important to successful implementation. It is virtually impossible to communicate too much or too often.

There are many proven ways to effectively communicate results. From the medical staff perspective, one of the best ways is to hold an evening medical staff meeting. In a typical meeting agenda, the president of the medical staff (a steering group member) kicks off the meeting with a brief overview of the clinical improvement program. Then the team leader of one of the pilot clinical improvement teams gives a review of the mission, the project team process, and the results. Through this brief presentation, the team shares with the medical staff the inside story of how TQM techniques combine applied scientific method, engineering methods, and good management to improve care to patients. Resolving chronic problems always sparks interest among clinicians. A question-and-answer period should follow.

After such a meeting a few more potential team leaders or participants will identify themselves. These physicians are intrigued by the concepts and the methodology and often express interest in receiving more training.

Another innovative approach is to expose all clinicians from a particular department or service together, setting the expectation for cross-functional initiatives. Communication strategies for non-physician clinicians and the remainder of the staff can follow a similar all-hands venue in the appropriate setting.

Another very successful communication tool is the use of storyboards, which are visual displays of the work of teams. They include the mission, the data collected, cause-and-effect analysis, interventions, and results achieved. These can be strategically positioned around the organization to stimulate interest and feedback from staff. Always consider the potential sensitivity of the data in selecting what, how, and where storyboards are displayed.

There is much for clinical leaders to do to implement a successful program.

### Tasks for Clinical Leaders During the Start Phase

- Support pilot projects teams.

  Training

  Time

  Resources

  Review

- Initiate infrastructure for quality improvement.

  Project process

  Reward and recognition

  Merit rating

  Training

  Resources

  Publicity and communications

- Establish assessments and measurements.

  Cost of poor quality

Market standing

Internal culture

Quality systems

At the end of the start phase the steering group conducts an annual review of its progress and updates the quality plan for the next phase.

## Phase 4: Expansion

Reaching this phase heralds to an organization that is beginning to emerge with a mature quality program. As the name implies, this phase essentially means expanding previous efforts. Organization units, number and types of teams, measurement, and training—all are expanded. At this phase TQM is no longer a program, it is a way of working as an organization and as individuals caring for patients.

### Expanded Organization Units

TQM now expands into more organization units. Divisions and departments create their own steering groups or quality councils, each with the same department-level responsibilities as the overall steering group has for the institution as a whole. These subordinate councils select their own projects, use facilitators to train department team members, write their own mission statements, provide resources, and empower these teams to fix problems and assess their results.

As long as the scope of their projects reside intradepartmentally, these teams may be required to provide only a brief summary of their activities to the main organizational steering group. If, however, these intradepartmental teams require resources beyond their departmental discretionary limits, they should be expected to take their data and their storyboards to the organizational steering group to advocate for reprioritization of resources.

## Expanded Teams

Across the entire organization a rapidly increasing number of teams, both interdepartmental and intradepartmental, arise as a result of expanding efforts to identify and address a myriad of chronic quality problems. The surgical department council may look at reducing deep-wound infection rates or creating a care path for total hip replacement. The medical department council may target length of stay for congestive heart failure. This proliferation will require an expanded capability to train facilitators, team leaders and team members.

The increase in types of teams also indicates organizational maturation. In addition to improvement teams, measurement (control) teams will evolve. Many of these will be clinical in nature and so will be led by clinicians. The measurement efforts will become even more sophisticated, will respond proactively to customer expectations, and will serve to strategically position the organization to be clinically competitive.

As measurement activities grow, the types of measures will be more closely tied to the organization's strategic plan. Outcome measures will more clearly reflect the target patient populations served by the organization. Topics will align with purchaser priorities. Time trend tracking of key indicators will be in place and reported to the steering group on a regular basis.

Moreover, at this time the organizational steering group should begin to look at the key business processes of the organization, processes so vital to the health of the organization that if they are not done correctly, it will not survive. Examples might be the admissions process, the discharge process, the intensive care process, and the referral process.

This may be the ideal time to charter and train a business process quality management team of senior-level people to work on reengineering one of these key business processes. For example, a team working to reengineer the intensive care process might include the following persons:

Intensive care medical director

Nursing head of the ICU

Chief of respiratory therapy

Senior surgeon

Senior medical intensivist

Supply department director

Inpatient pharmacy director

## Expanded Training

The training requirements will expand as well. In addition to facilitators, team leaders, and team members, all middle managers or supervisors will require more training in concepts such as empowerment and quality in daily work. This training allows the supervisors to train their own departments, establish their own councils, write mission statements, and assist in team training—in other words, to bring quality management to the people closest to the processes.

Senior clinical managers will likewise require advanced training in areas such as benchmarking. This is the work of identifying best demonstrated practices, studying the processes that yield the best results, and subsequently exceeding the benchmark performance. For example, a surgical team desiring to improve deep-wound infection rates might visit Intermountain Health Care, study the processes used to achieve best-practice infection rates, then return home to implement improvements designed to improve those rates even beyond those achieved by Intermountain Health Care.

As leaders become more comfortable with the use of quality tools and principles, it is expected that they would perform more of the subordinate teaching required during the expand phase. Nothing sends a louder, clearer, more positive message than clinical leaders themselves teaching TQM.

Much of the important senior leadership training will come from the steering group seeing itself as a learning body. They should set aside time so that members can share insights gathered from books and journals, conferences, and other learning experiences. This self-education is vital and should be a routine component of leadership meetings.

*Tasks for Clinical Leaders During the Expansion Phase*

- Support quality infrastructure.

- Support expansion of teams.

- Participate in training.

- Participate in projects.

- Charter quality improvement teams.

- Charter quality planning teams.

- Charter expansion of quality measurement.

- Identify key business processes.

- Create key business process teams.

- Lead the strategic quality planning (see Chapter Seven).

Clearly, the tasks facing clinical leaders during the expand phase of TQM implementation are considerable. Success of TQM during this challenging phase rests heavily on the ability of clinical leaders to take charge, to collaborate closely with administrative leadership (especially on the organization's steering group and councils at all levels), and to constantly model and reinforce the new management approach.

## Phase 5: Integration

Experts in quality management say it takes six to ten years for an organization to fully enculturate TQM. Why so long? Pilot teams, benchmarking, strategic planning, and other techniques can be introduced into an organization in a much shorter time.

The integration phase demonstrates why it takes this length of time for TQM to become a way of life. During this phase (see Figure 8.1), goals, people, key business processes, and reviews and audits are interwoven and fully integrated so that the organization's focus is directed toward making the vision a reality. All staff and employees participate on teams in some way. This can happen only when clinical leaders are fully involved and committed.

**Integrating Goals**

Goal integration requires that the organizational-level strategic goals (including those specifically focused on patient groups and diagnosis) cascade down to the cross-functional, the departmental, and the individual level.

For example, consider the strategic goal to become a world-class women's health care program. To make this a reality, cross-functional goals between primary care and oncology regarding breast cancer screening, diagnosis, and treatment are achieved by

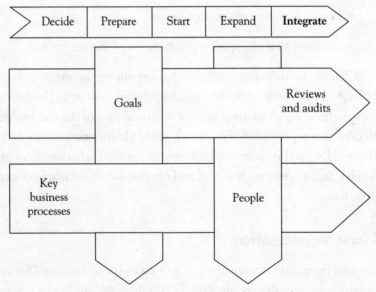

Figure 8.1. The Integrated Organization.

design, improvement, and measurement teams. The same process operates for other major health concerns of women. For example, the department of obstetrics and gynecology implements department goals to support this element of the key organization strategy for obstetrical care. Furthermore, individual clinicians and support technicians establish individual goals to ensure departmental goal achievement. An obstetrician might, for example, set an individual goal of ensuring 100 percent of the patient population between fifty and sixty-five have screening mammograms, if indicated. Individual goals are the building blocks of departmental, cross-functional, and strategic organizational goals and success.

**Integrating People**

Individuals' efforts must likewise be fully integrated with an overall organizational plan. To begin with, the appropriate level of training must be planned. Everyone will require training in the appropriate areas to ensure organizational success. This training includes:

- Team facilitation

- Team leadership

- Applied epidemiology

- Patient-focused care

- Outcomes measurement

- Team member participation

- Business process quality management

- Benchmarking

- Self-directed work teams

- Strategic quality planning

Next, the question of empowerment must be addressed. Health care reform threatens to take power out of the hands of the clinician. Critical to the success of the integration phase is the clinicians' realization that they are empowered. They negotiate with purchasers to come to consensus on what should be measured. They analyze measures and identify opportunities for improvement. They lead member improvement and care pathway teams. They monitor the improved levels of patient care. They are key players in the use of benchmarking, strategic quality planning, and other TQM tools. They can dramatically affect market standing of their organizations as a result of their participation in TQM activities.

Finally, steps must be taken to enhance teamwork, which is critical to the integration phase. In particular, clinicians and administrators working collaboratively on measurement teams, improvement teams, care pathway teams, and benchmarking teams create an atmosphere of trust and collegiality in which everyone, including the patient, wins.

## Integrating Business Processes

Key business processes are now fully integrated. The critical success factors for the organization are identified. Key business processes are identified. Process owners are assigned and teams set up to measure and optimize the performance of these vital functions. Teams are trained, results are measured, and findings integrated into processes.

Many of these key business processes require clinician participation at all phases of measurement and improvement because they involve areas in which only clinicians have a full understanding of process performance. For example, the vice president for operations is the key stakeholder for the admissions process. In order to reengineer this key process, goals must be set for cycle times and patient flow. Clinicians are involved on this reengineering team. Specifically, they contribute to the understanding of clinician involvement in the current process and, more important, how the process can be streamlined from the clinician's perspective.

### Integrating Reviews and Audits

Integration would not be complete without ongoing reviews and audits. It is important that market standing undergo continual analysis. Clinicians assist by providing input concerning their knowledge of comparative and competitive performance. Clinicians affiliated with multiple organizations can provide important insight on how one organization compares to another.

The ongoing assessments of costs of poor quality reveal opportunities to improve care and reduce waste. Annual questionnaires and interviews designed to update understanding of the internal culture of the organization validate that change is happening and that the organization is moving in the right direction. Specifically, clinicians are surveyed on how process improvements are impacting their practices, how team activities are achieving desired results, and how collaboration makes practice more rewarding.

Likewise, as the quality system of councils, facilitators, key business process teams, and inter- and intradepartmental teams continues to evolve, clinicians and their leaders play a vital role of leadership, mentoring, and participation.

Finally, results of reviews and audits by organizations such as the JCAHO, the NCQA, the College of American Pathologists, and the Healthplan Employer Data and Information Set (HEDIS) require analysis and action. Clinicians are critical to the success of an organization's reaction to these mandates.

Figure 8.2 summarizes the various elements of the integration model, and the following list summarizes the tasks that clinical leaders must perform during this final yet never-ending phase.

*Tasks for Clinical Leaders During the Integration Phase*

- Integrate quality goals into the business plan.

- Deploy action to units and cross-functional teams.

- Act on audits of quality systems.

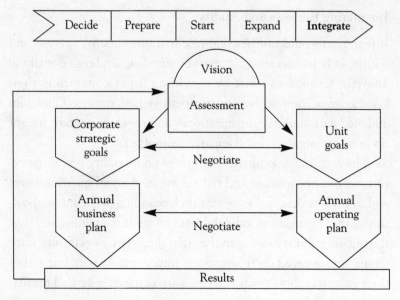

Figure 8.2. The Integration Model.

- Integrate cross-functional process measures and results.

- Charter unit quality assessments.

- Charter and support training for all.

- Enable full employee participation with training and resources.

- Expand personal participation in quality.

## Conclusion

Experience with numerous health care organizations that have achieved astounding successes in TQM serves to validate the importance that clinical leaders play during each successive phase. These agents of change are defining health care reform at its most basic, grassroots level.

# Conclusion

. . . . . . . . . . . . . . . . . . . . . . . . . . . . . .

# Panacea, Placebo, or the Right Prescription?

With all the pressure for change in health care, the stresses on physicians make practicing medicine more challenging than ever before. There is tension between practitioners, specialties, and organizations. The rate of change is astounding. The question foremost in the minds of health professionals today is: In the midst of all this, how do I cope, compete, and, with any luck, find day-to-day personal gratification in my work?

Where does quality management fit in? Is it a panacea or a placebo? How should it be viewed? From the experience of many organizations, there are some key lessons to making a management strategy work that can help to answer these questions.

First, recognize that effective solutions call for fundamental change in the way organizations approach all aspects of professionalism and business. Some have used the term *paradigm shift* to imply changes of major proportion. Changes of this magnitude cannot occur overnight. It is crucial to recognize that this is a long-term commitment.

A second key lesson is to realize that leaders must acquire new knowledge, skills, and behaviors. For most people, implementing a successful strategy requires significant new learning. Again, this means making a personal investment of time and attention over months and years.

A third and related lesson is to minimize the religiosity and jargon in your program. If TQM is presented as a panacea, it will likely function as a placebo, at best. The impact will be temporary. It will be rejected as superficial and will certainly fail. It is important to be honest about individual organizations and their current state, noting that change is by and large incremental.

Finally, and perhaps most important, maintain an awareness and openness about how organizations manage quality and cost. The success stories are still new and there are many lessons yet to be learned. No organization has all the answers at this stage. Even cutting-edge leaders in health care are still finding their way. The American health care system will look radically different in a decade. Both financing and delivery system organization will undergo extraordinary change during the next few years. Any particular organization that survives will have found an approach, methods, and techniques for achieving outstanding results and innovation.

Total quality management offers an approach and techniques that health care organizations can use to achieve their goals. It is certainly not a panacea. If it is implemented as a quick fix, it will only frustrate and alienate clinicians. TQM is not a religion, rather it is both an art and a science. At the same time, TQM is not a placebo; the problems facing health care organizations are far too great for any superficial solution.

TQM does require hard work and diligence, a willingness to try, fail, and try again. Just like the study and practice of medicine, the investment pays off in both measurable and immeasurable ways.

# References

American Health Consultants. "Why Alliant and Toronto Hospitals Are Reassessing Hundreds of Paths." *Hospital Case Management*, 1993, *1*(3), 41–45.

American Medical Association. *Directory of Practice Parameters*. Chicago: American Medical Association, 1992.

Andersson, S. "Quality Planning for Clinical Processes of Care." *Quality Letter*, 1993, *5*(5), 2–4.

Angelo, L. J., and Sokol, R. J. "Short- Versus Long-Course Prophylactic Antibiotic Treatment in Cesarean Section Patients." *Obstetrics and Gynecology*, 1980, *55*, 583–586.

Armstrong, D. "General Practitioners' View of Clinical Guidelines for the Management of Asthma." *International Journal for Quality in Health Care*, 1994, *6*(2), 199–202.

Arvantes, J. C. "Using TQM to Forge Customer-Driven Strategic Planning." *Quality Letter*, 1993, *5*(10), 11–14.

Bader, B. "Capitation Payment: How Fee-for-Service Medicine Is Making the Transition." *Quality Letter*, 1993a, *5*(4), 2–12.

Bader, B. "Quality Improvement in Action: Second Annual Issue." *Quality Letter*, 1993b, *5*(1), 1–32.

Barnes, R., Lawton, L., and Briggs, D. "Clinical Benchmarking Improves Clinical Paths: Experience with Coronary Artery Bypass Grafting." *Journal on Quality Improvement*, 1994, *20*(5), 267–274.

Barton, M. B., and Schoenbaum, S. C. "Improving Influenza Vaccine Performance in an HMO Setting: The Use of Computer-Generated Reminders and Peer Comparison Feedback." *American Journal of Public Health*, 1990, *80*, 534–536.

Berman, S. (ed.). "Making Good on the Promise: Disseminating and Implementing Practice Guidelines." *Quality Review Bulletin*, 1992, *18*(12), 393–482.

Berwick, D. M. "Controlling Variation in Health Care: A Consultation with Walter Shewhart." *Medical Care*, 1991, *29*(12), 1212–1225.

Bloomberg, M. "Development of Clinical Indicators for Performance Measurement and Improvement: An HMO/Purchase Collaborative Effort." *Journal on Quality Improvement*, 1993, *19*(12), 586–598.

Cafasso, E. "Hospitals Abused Medicare." *Boston Herald*, June 24, 1992.

Caldwell, C. Personal communication. 1994.

Campbell, A. B. "Scripps Health System." Presentation at the Power of Quality conference sponsored by the Health Care Forum, San Diego, Calif., June 1993a.

Campbell, A. B. "Strategic Planning in Health Care: Methods and Applications." *Quality Management in Health Care*, 1993b, *1*(4), 12–13.

Campbell, A. B. "Benchmarking: A Performance Intervention Tool." *Journal on Quality Improvement*, 1994, *20*(5), 225–228.

Classen, D. C., Evans, S. R., and Pestonik, S. L. "The Timing of Prophylactic Administration of Antibiotics and the Risk of Surgical Wound Infection." *New England Journal of Medicine*, 1992, *326*(5), 281–286.

Coffey, R. J., and others. "An Introduction to Critical Paths." *Quality Management in Health Care*, 1992, *1*(1), 45–54.

Collaborative Group on Preterm Birth. "Multicenter Randomized Controlled Trial of a Preterm Birth Prevention Program." *American Journal of Obstetrics and Gynecology*, 1993, *169*(2), 362–366.

Collins, K., Quinlan, A., Farrell, M., and Snyder, L. M. "Influencing Physician Behavior with CQI: A Case Study." *Quality Management in Health Care*, 1994, *2*(3), 27–35.

Conrad, D. A., and Dowling, W. "Vertical Integration in Health Services: Theory and Management Implications." *Health Care Management Review*, 1990, *15*(4), 9–22.

Corrigan, J., and Nielson, D. "Toward the Development of Uniform Reporting Standards for Managed Care Organizations: The Health Plan Employer Data and Information Set, Version 2.0." *Journal on Quality Improvement*, 1993, *19*(12), 566–575.

Cox, S. M., and Gilstrap, L. C. "Postpartum Endometritis." *Clinical Obstetrics and Gynecology*, 1989, *16*(2), 363–371.

Crosby, P. B. *Quality Is Free: The Art of Making Quality Certain.* New York: McGraw-Hill, 1979.

Curtis, L. H. (ed.). *Quality Measurement and Management Initiative Coronary Revascularization Project Protocol* (version 2.0). Rochester, N.Y.: Academic Medical Center Consortium, 1994.

Dalkey, N. C., and Helmer, O. *An Experimental Application of the Delphi Method to the Use of Experts.* (Publication No. RM727PR.) Chicago: Rand Corp., 1967.

Davis, B. "The Prevention Guidelines from Group Health Cooperative of Puget Sound." In N. Goldfield, M. Pine, and J. Pine (eds.), *Measuring and Managing Health Care Quality: Procedures, Techniques, and Protocols.* Gaithersburg, Md.: Aspen, 1991.

Delbanco, T. L. "Enriching the Doctor-Patient Relationship by Inviting the Patient's Perspective." *Annals of Internal Medicine,* 1992, *116*(5), 414–417.

Delbecq, A. *Group Techniques for Program Planning: A Guide to Nominal Group and Delphi Processes.* Chicago: Scott, Foresman, 1975.

Deming, W. E. *Out of Crisis.* Cambridge, Mass.: Center for Advanced Engineering Study, Massachusetts Institute of Technology, 1986.

De Mott, K. "Critical Pathways Save $6.4 Million, Cut ALOS at the Christ Hospital." *Report on Medical Guidelines and Outcomes Research,* 1994, *5*(18), 1–5.

Dick, R. S., and Steen, E. B. (eds.). *The Computer-Based Patient Record: An Essential Technology for Health Care.* Washington, D.C.: National Academy Press, 1991.

Donabedian, A. "The End Results of Health Care: Ernest Codman's Contribution to Quality Assessment and Beyond." *Milbank Quarterly,* 1989, *67*(2), 233–256.

Donowitz, L. G., and Wenzel, R. P. "Endometritis Following Cesarean Section: A Controlled Study of the Increased Duration of Hospital Stay and Direct Cost of Hospitalization." *American Journal of Obstetrics and Gynecology,* 1980, *137*(4), 467–469.

Eddy, D. M. "Designing a Practice Policy: Standards, Guidelines, and Options." *Journal of the American Medical Association,* 1990a, *263*(22), 3077–3084.

Eddy, D. M. "Guidelines for Policy Statements: The Explicit Approach." *Journal of the American Medical Association,* 1990b, *263*(16), 2239–2243.

Eddy, D. M. *A Manual for Assessing Health Practices and Designing Practice Policies: The Explicit Approach.* Philadelphia: American College of Physicians, 1992.

Eddy, D. M., and Billings, J. "The Quality of Medical Evidence: Implications for Quality Care." *Health Affairs,* 1988, *7*(19), 19–32.

Eraker, S. "Understanding and Improving Patient Compliance." *Annals of Internal Medicine,* 1984, *100*(2), 258–268.

Falconer, J. A., and others. "The Critical Path Method in Stroke Rehabilitation: Lessons from an Experiment in Cost Containment and Outcome Improvement." *Quality Review Bulletin*, 1993, *19*(1), 8–15.

Field, M. J., and Lohr, K. N. *Guidelines for Clinical Practice: From Development to Use.* Washington, D.C.: National Academy Press, 1992.

Fink, A., Kosecoff, J., Chassin, M., and Brook, R. H. "Consensus Methods: Characteristics and Guidelines for Use." *American Journal of Public Health*, 1984, *74*(9), 979–983.

Gall, S., and others. "Beneficial Effects of Endotracheal Extubation on Ventricular Performance." *Journal of Thoracic and Cardiovascular Surgery*, 1988, *95*(5), 819–827.

Gaucher, E. J., and Coffey, R. J. *Total Quality in Healthcare: From Theory to Practice.* San Francisco: Jossey-Bass, 1993.

Goal/QPC. *The Memory Jogger: A Pocket Guide of Tools for Continuous Improvement.* (2nd ed.) Methuen, Mass.: Goal/QPC, 1988.

Goldfield, N., and Nash, D. B. (eds.). *Providing Quality Care: The Challenge to Physicians.* Philadelphia: American College of Physicians, 1989.

Goldfield, N., Pine, M., and Pine, J. (eds.). *Measuring and Managing Health Care Quality: Procedures, Techniques, and Protocols.* Gaithersburg, Md.: Aspen, 1991.

Goodwin, D. R. "Critical Pathways in Home Health Care." *Journal of Nursing Administration*, 1992, *22*(2), 34–40.

Gottlieb, L. K., Sokol, N., Murray, K., and Schoenbaum, S. C. "Algorithm-Based Clinical Quality Improvement." *HMO Practice*, 1992, *6*(1), 5–12.

Greco, P. J., and Eisenberg, J. "Changing Physicians' Practices." *New England Journal of Medicine*, 1993, *329*(17), 1271–1274.

Greenfield, S., and Nelson, E. C. "Recent Developments and Future Issues in the Use of Health Status Assessment Measures in Clinical Settings." *Medical Care*, 1992, *30*(5), MS23–MS41.

Greenfield, S., and others. "Patient Participation in Medical Care: Effects on Blood Sugar Control and Quality of Life in Diabetes." *Journal of General Internal Medicine*, 1988, *3*(5), 448–457.

Grilli, R., and Lomas, J. "Evaluating the Message: The Relationships Between Compliance Rate and the Subject of a Practice Guideline." *Medical Care*, 1994, *32*(3), 202–213.

Guadagnoli, E., and McNeil, B. J. "Outcomes Research: Hope for the Future or the Latest Rage?" *Inquiry*, 1994, *31*(1), 14–24.

Gustafson, D., Taylor, J., Thompson, S., and Chesney, P. "Assessing the Needs of Breast Cancer Patients and Their Families." *Quality Management in Health Care*, 1993, *2*(1), 6–17.

Handley, M. R., Stuart, M., and Kirz, H. "Evidence-Based Approach to Evaluating and Improving Clinical Practice: Implementing Practice Guidelines." *HMO Practice*, 1994, 8(2), 75–83.

Hofmann, P. "Critical Path Method: An Important Tool for Coordinating Clinical Care." *Journal on Quality Improvement*, 1993, 19(7), 235–246.

Iezzoni, L. I. "Measuring Severity of Illness and Casemix." In N. Goldfield and D. B. Nash (eds.), *Providing Quality Care: The Challenge to Physicians*. Philadelphia: American College of Physicians, 1989.

Iezzoni, L. I. "Severity Standardization and Hospital Quality Assessment." In J. B. Couch (ed.), *Health Care Quality Management for the 21st Century*. Tampa, Fla.: American College of Physician Executives, 1991.

Iezzoni, L. I. "Choosing a Severity Measure" (editorial). *American College of Medical Quality*, 1994a, 9(3), 101–115.

Iezzoni, L. I. "Identify Complications of Care Using Administrative Data." *Medical Care*, 1994b, 32(7), 700–715.

Iezzoni, L. I. (ed). *Risk Adjustment for Measuring Health Care Outcomes*. Ann Arbor, Mich.: Health Administration Press, 1994c.

Iezzoni, L. I. "Using Administrative Data to Screen Hospitals for High Complication Rate." *Inquiry*, 1994d, 31(1), 40–52.

Iezzoni, L. I., and Daly, J. "A Description and Clinical Assessment of the Computerized Severity Index." *Quality Review Bulletin*, 1992, 18(2), 44–52.

Iezzoni, L. I., and Moskowitz, M. A. "A Clinical Assessment of MedisGroups." *Journal of the American Medical Association*, 1988, 260(21), 3159–3163.

Institute of Medicine. *Preventing Low Birth Weight*. Washington, D.C.: National Academy Press, 1985.

Institute of Medicine. *Medicare: A Strategy for Quality Assurance*. (vol. 1). Ed. K. N. Lohr. Washington, D.C.: National Academy Press, 1990.

Ishikawa, K. *Guide to Quality Control*. White Plains, N.Y.: Kraus International, 1982.

James, B. *Quality Management in Health Care Delivery*. Chicago: Hospital Research and Education Trust, 1989.

James, B., Horn, S., and Stephenson, R. "Management by Fact: What Is CPI and How Is It Used?" In S. Horn and D. S. Hopkins (eds.), *Clinical Practice Improvement*. Washington, D.C.: Faulkner and Gray, 1994.

Jennison Goonan, K. A. "Employers' Expectations for Information on Quality." *HMO/PPO Trends*, 1991, 5(4), 7–12.

Jennison Goonan, K. A., and Jordan, H. "Is Quality Assurance Antiquated, or Was It at the Right Place at the Wrong Time?" *Quality Review Bulletin*, 1992, 18(11), 372–379.

Johnson, T. F. "Asthma Home Care Program." Unpublished report. Andover, Mass., 1992.

Joint Commission on Accreditation of Healthcare Organizations. *Primer on Indicator Development and Applications*. Oakbrook Terrace, Ill.: Joint Commission on Accreditation of Healthcare Organizations, 1990.

Joint Commission on Accreditation of Healthcare Organizations. *Using CQI Approaches to Monitor, Evaluate, and Improve Quality*. Oakbrook Terrace, Ill.: Joint Commission on Accreditation of Healthcare Organizations, 1991.

Joint Commission on Accreditation of Healthcare Organizations. *Development and Application of Indicators of Emergency Care*. Oakbrook Terrace, Ill.: Joint Commission on Accreditation of Healthcare Organizations, 1993a.

Joint Commission on Accreditation of Healthcare Organizations. *The Measurement Mandate*. Oakbrook Terrace, Ill.: Joint Commission on Accreditation of Healthcare Organizations, 1993b.

Joyce, T., Corman, H., and Grossman, M. "A Cost-Effectiveness Analysis of Strategies to Reduce Infant Mortality." *Medical Care*, 1988, 26(4), 348–360.

Juran, J. M. *Juran on Planning for Quality*. New York: Free Press, 1988.

Juran, J. M. *Juran on Leadership for Quality*. New York: Free Press, 1989.

Juran, J. M., and Gryna, F. M. (eds.). *Juran's Quality Control Handbook*. (4th ed.). New York: McGraw-Hill, 1988.

Juran Institute. *Quality Improvement in Health Care: Facilitator's Tool Kit*. Wilton, Conn.: Juran Institute, 1993a.

Juran Institute. *Strategic Quality Planning*. Wilton, Conn.: Juran Institute, 1993b.

Kaplan, S. H., and Ware, J. E. "The Patient's Role in Health Care and Quality Assessment." In N. Goldfield and D. B. Nash (eds.), *Providing Quality Care: The Challenge to Physicians*. Philadelphia: American College of Physicians, 1989.

Kassirer, J. "The Quality of Care and the Quality of Measuring It." *New England Journal of Medicine*, 1993, 329(17), 1263–1265.

Kassirer, J. "The Use and Abuse of Practice Profiles." *New England Journal of Medicine*, 1994, 330(9), 634–635.

Kelly, J., and Toepp, M. C. "Practice Parameters: Development, Evaluation, Dissemination, and Implementation." *Quality Review Bulletin*, 1992, 18(12), 405–409.

Klineberg, P., Geer, R., Hirsh, R., and Aukburg, S. "Early Extubation After Bypass Graft Surgery." *Critical Care Medicine*, 1977, 5(6), 272–274.

Kosecoff, J., and others. "Effects of the National Institutes of Health Consensus Development Program on Physician Practice." *Journal of the American Medical Association*, 1987, 258(19), 2708–2713.

Kritchevsky, S. B., and Simmons, B. P. "Continuous Quality Improvement: Concepts and Applications for Physician Care." *Journal of the American Medical Association*, 1991, 266(13), 1817–1823.

Lanman, R. B. "Improving Pediatric Asthma Care in a Health Maintenance Organization." In S. Horn and D. S. Hopkins (eds.), *Clinical Practice Improvement.* Washington, D.C.: Faulkner and Gray, 1994.

Letsch, S. W., and others. "National Health Expenditures." *Health Care Financial Review,* 1992, *14*(2), 1–30.

Lomas, J. "Do Practice Guidelines Guide Practice? The Effect of a Consensus Statement on the Practice of Physicians." *New England Journal of Medicine,* 1989, *321*(19), 1306–1311.

Lomas, J., and Haynes, R. B. "A Taxonomy and Critical Review of Vested Strategies for the Application of Clinical Practice Recommendations: From 'Official' to 'Individual' Clinical Policy." *American Journal of Preventive Medicine,* 1988, *4*(4), 77–94.

Lomas, J., and others. "Opinion Leaders vs. Audit and Feedback to Implement Guidelines: Delivery After Previous Cesarean Section." *Journal of the American Medical Association,* 1991, *265*(17), 2202–2207.

Luttman, R. J. "The Critical Path Method Alone Does Nothing to Improve Performance." *Quality Review Bulletin,* 1993, *19*(5), 142–143.

Lynch, J. "The 'Toward Excellence in Care' Program: A Statewide Indicator Project." *Journal on Quality Management,* 1993, *19*(11), 519–529.

McGarvey, R. N., and Harper, J. J. "Pneumonia Mortality Reduction and Quality Improvement in a Community Hospital." *Quality Review Bulletin,* 1993, *19*(5), 124–130.

McNeil, B. J., Pedersen, S. H., and Gatsonis, C. "Current Issues in Profiles: Potentials and Limitations." In *Conference on Profiling.* (Publication No. 92–2). Washington, D.C.: Physician Payment Review Commission, 1992.

Mandelker, J. "Government Purchasers See Value in Managed Care." *Business and Health,* 1993, *11*(8), 40–42, 44.

Markson, L. E., and Nash, D. B. "Quality and Accountability." *Journal on Quality Improvement,* 1994, *20*(7), 353–418.

Mitka, M. "Managed Care and Business to Develop Clinical 'Report Card.'" *American Medical News,* Feb. 8, 1993, p. 15.

Mugford, M., Banfield, P., and O'Hanlon, M. "Effects of Feedback of Information on Clinical Practice: A Review." *British Medical Journal,* 1991, *303*(6799), 398–402.

Mulley, A. F., and Eagle, K. A. "What Is Appropriate Care?" *Journal of the American Medical Association,* 1988, *260*(4), 540–541.

Nadzam, D. "Data-Driven Performance Improvement in Health Care: The Joint Commission's Indicator Measurement System." *Journal on Quality Improvement,* 1991, *19*(11), 492–500.

National Committee on Quality Assurance. *Standards for Managed Care Accreditation*. Washington, D.C.: National Committee on Quality Assurance, 1994.

National Heart, Lung and Blood Institute. *Executive Summary Guidelines for the Diagnosis and Management of Asthma*. (Publication No. HIH 91–3042A.) Bethesda, Md.: National Heart, Lung and Blood Institute, 1991.

Nelson, E. C., and Batalden, P. B. "Patient-Based Quality Measurement Systems." *Quality Management in Health Care*, 1993, *2*(1), 18–31.

Nelson, E. C., and Wasson, J. H. "Using Patient-Based Information to Rapidly Redesign Care." *Health Care Forum Journal*, July-Aug. 1993, pp. 25–29.

Nerenz, D. R. "Consortium Research on Indicators of System Performance (CRISP)." *Journal on Quality Improvement*, 1993, *19*(12), 577–585.

O'Leary, D. S., and Schyve, P. "The Role of Accreditation in Quality Oversight and Improvement Under Health Care Reform." *Quality Letter*, 1993, *5*(10), 11–14.

O'Reilly, P. "On Disclosure of Quality of Care Data." Conference proceedings, Massachusetts Peer Review Organization, Waltham, Dec. 1, 1993.

Pennsylvania Cost Containment Council. *Coronary Artery Bypass Graft Surgery: A Technical Report*. Harrisburg: Pennsylvania Cost Containment Council, 1992.

Platt, R. "Harvard Community Health Plan Mammography Screening Project." *Quality Connection*, 1991, *1*(1), 12–13.

Plsek, P. *Quality Improvement Tools*. Wilton, Conn.: Juran Institute, 1989.

Quasha, A., and others. "Postoperative Respiratory Care: A Controlled Trial of Early Extubation and Late Extubation Following Coronary Bypass Grafting." *Anesthesiology*, 1989, *52*(2), 135–141.

Quill, T. "Recognizing and Adjusting to Barriers in Doctor-Patient Communication." *Annals of Internal Medicine*, 1989, *111*(1), 51–58.

Ramsay, J. G., and others. "Early Extubation After High-Dose Fentanyl Anesthesia for Aortocoronary Bypass Surgery: Reversal of Respiratory Depression with Low-Dose Nalbuphine." *Canadian Anaesthetists Society Journal*, 1985, *32*(6), 597–605.

Relman, A. S. "Assessment and Accountability: The Third Revolution in Medical Care." *New England Journal of Medicine*, 1988, *319*(18), 1220–1222.

Rolnick, S. J., Madden, J., Stukel, J., and Kopher, R. "Decrease in the Rate of Ruptured Ectopic Pregnancies: A Successful Team Approach." *HMO Practice*, 1994, *8*(3), 105–107.

Roper, W., Winkenwerder, W., Hackbarth, G., and Krakauer, H. "Effectiveness in Healthcare." *New England Journal of Medicine*, 1988, *319*(18), 1197–1202.

Ross, P. J. *Taguchi Techniques for Quality Engineering*. New York: McGraw-Hill, 1988.

Schlackman, N. "Integrating Quality Assessment and Physician Incentive Payment." *Quality Review Bulletin*, 1989, *15*(8), 235–238.

Schneider, M. (ed.). *Health Pages, St. Louis*. St. Louis: Health Pages, 1993.

Schoenbaum, S. C. "Feedback of Clinical Performance Information." *HMO Practice*, 1993, *7*(1), 5–11.

Schoenbaum, S. C., and Gottlieb, L. K. "Algorithm-Based Improvement of Clinical Quality." *British Medical Journal*, 1990, *301*(6765), 1374–1376.

Scholtes, P. R., and others. *The Team Handbook*. Madison, Wis.: Joiner Associates, 1988.

Schriefer, J. "Reducing the Length of Stay for Postoperative Open-Heart Patients." *Quality Connection*, 1993, *2*(3), 8–9.

Schriefer, J. "The Synergy of Pathways and Algorithms: Two Tools Work Better Than One." *Journal on Quality Improvement*, 1994, *20*(9), 485–499.

Schyve, P. "Setting Priorities for Improvement." *Quality Letter*, 1994, *6*(4), 33.

Sennett, C., Legorreta, A., and Zatz, S. "Performance-Based Hospital Contracting for Quality Improvement." *Joint Commission Journal on Continuous Improvement*, 1993, *19*(9), 374–383.

Shaller, D. V., Pine, M., Naessens, J., and Ballard, D. "Greater Cost-Effectiveness in Health Care Delivery." *Group Practice Journal*, Jan. 1992.

Shewhart, W. A. *Statistical Method from the Viewpoint of Quality Control*. Milwaukee, Wis.: Quality Press, 1986. (Originally published in 1939.)

Siu, A., and others. "Choosing Quality of Care Measures Based on Expected Impact of Improved Care on Health." *Health Services Research*, 1992, *27*(5), 619–650.

Smith, R., and Hoppe, R. "The Patient's Story: Integrating the Patient and Physician-Centered Approaches to Interviewing." *Annals of Internal Medicine*, 1991, *115*(6), 470–477.

Stein, C. "A Mixed Bag for Mass. Health Insurers." *Boston Globe*, Mar. 17, 1994.

Stump, M. A. "Minnesota Blue Cross and Blue Shield." Presentation at the Capture, Navigation, and Use Health Data Information Strategy Conference, Institute for International Research, Boston, July 1993.

SunHealth Alliance. *Self-Assessment of Healthcare Organizational Performance*. Charlotte, N.C.: SunHealth Alliance, 1994.

Tierney, W. M., Hui, S. L., and McDonald, C. J. "Delayed Feedback of Physicians Performance vs. Immediate Reminders to Perform Preventive Care: Effects on Physician Compliance." *Medical Care*, 1986, *24*(8), 659–666.

Townsend, P. L., with Gebhart, J. E. *Commit to Quality*. New York: Wiley, 1990.

Van Amringe, M., and Shannon, T. "Awareness, Assimilation, and Adoption: The Challenge of Effective Dissemination and the First AHCPR-Sponsored Guidelines." *Quality Review Bulletin*, 1992, *18*(12), 397–404.

Veatch, R. "Integrating TQM and Strategic Planning." *Quality Letter*, 1993, *5*(7), 1.

Vibbert, S., Migdail, K. J., Strickland, D., and Youngs, M. T. *The Medical Outcomes and Guideline Sourcebook*. Washington, D.C.: Faulker and Gray, 1994.

Walton, M. *The Deming Management Method*. New York: Putnam, 1986.

Weingarten, S., and Ellrodt, A. G. "The Case for Intensive Dissemination: Adoption of Practice Guidelines in the Coronary Care Unit." *Quality Review Bulletin*, 1992, *18*(12), 449–455.

Weingarten, S., and others. "Early Stepdown Transfer of Low-Risk Patients with Chest Pain." *Annals of Internal Medicine*, 1990, *113*(4), 283–289.

Weingarten, S., and others. "Practice Guidelines and Reminders to Reduce Duration of Hospital Stay for Patients with Chest Pain." *Annals of Internal Medicine*, 1994, *120*(4), 247–263.

Wennberg, J. E. "Which Rate Is Right?" *New England Journal of Medicine*, 1986, *314*(5), 310–311.

Wheeler, D. J. *Understanding Variation: The Key to Managing Chaos*. Knoxville, Tenn.: SPC Press, 1993.

Wickizer, T. "The Effect of Utilization Review on Hospital Use and Expenditures." In T. Grannemann (ed.), *Review, Regulate, or Reform: What Works to Control Workers Compensation Medical Costs*. Cambridge, Mass.: Workers Compensation Research Institute, 1994.

Willard, J. E., Lange, R. A., and Hillis, L. D. "The Use of Aspirin in Ischemic Health Disease." *New England Journal of Medicine*, 1992, *327*(3), 175–181.

Williams, S., Nash, D. B., and Goldfield, N. "Differences in Mortality from Coronary Artery Bypass Graft Surgery at Five Teaching Hospitals." *Journal of the American Medical Association*, 1991, *266*(6), 810.

Winslow, R. "Medicare Tries to Save with One-Fee Billing for Some Operations." *Wall Street Journal*, June 10, 1992.

Wise, D. "HMO Ratings Spur Quality Efforts." *Business and Health*, 1994, *12*(9), 65–66.

Zander, K. "Care Maps: The Core of Cost/Quality Care." *The New Definition*, 1991, *6*(3), 1–3.

# Recommended Reading

Berwick, D. M. "Continuous Improvement As an Ideal in Health Care." *New England Journal of Medicine*, 1989, *320*, 53–56.

Berwick, D. M., Godfrey, A. B., and Roessner, J. *Curing Health Care: New Strategies for Quality Improvement*. San Francisco: Jossey-Bass, 1990.

Brassard, M. *The Memory Jogger Plus: Featuring the Seven Management and Planning Tools*. Methuen, Mass.: Goal/QPC, 1989.

Eddy, D. M. *A Manual for Assessing Health Practices and Designing Practice Policies: The Explicit Approach*. Philadelphia: American College of Physicians, 1992.

Eisenberg, J. M. *Doctors' Decisions and the Cost of Medical Care*. Ann Arbor, Mich.: Health Administration Press, 1986.

Gaucher, E. J., and Coffey, R. J. *Total Quality in Healthcare: From Theory to Practice*. San Francisco: Jossey-Bass, 1993.

Goal/QPC. *The Memory Jogger: A Pocket Guide of Tools for Continuous Improvement*. (2nd ed.). Methuen, Mass.: Goal/QPC.

Joint Commission on Accreditation of Healthcare Organizations. *Striving Toward Improvement: Six Hospitals in Search of Quality*. Oakbrook Terrace, Ill.: Joint Commission on Accreditation of Healthcare Organizations, 1992.

Juran, H. M. *Juran on Planning for Quality*. New York: Free Press, 1988.

Juran, H. M. *Juran on Leadership for Quality*. New York: Free Press, 1989.

Juran Institute. *Total Quality Management: A Practical Guide*. Wilton, Conn.: Juran Institute, 1991.

Scherkenbach, W. W. *The Deming Route to Quality and Productivity: Road Maps and Roadblocks*. Washington, D.C.: CEEP Press Books, 1988.

Scholtes, P. R., and others. *The Team Handbook*. Madison, Wis.: Joiner Associates, 1988.

Townsend, P. L., with Gebhart, J. E. *Commit to Quality*. New York: Wiley, 1990.

## Recommended Journals

*Hospital Case Management.* American Health Consultants, Atlanta.

*Joint Commission Perspectives.* Joint Commission on Accreditation of Healthcare Organizations, Oakbrook Terrace, Ill.

*Managed Care Medicine.* Health Care Communications, Fort Lee, N.J.

*Medical Outcomes and Guidelines Alert.* Faulkner and Gray's Healthcare Information Center, Washington, D.C.

*The Quality Connection.* Institute for Healthcare Improvement, Boston.

*The Quality Letter for Healthcare Leaders.* Bader & Associates, Rockville, Md.

*Report on Medical Guidelines and Outcomes Research.* Capitol Publications, Alexandria, Va.

*Strategies for Healthcare Excellence.* COR Healthcare Resources, Santa Barbara, Calif.

# Index